Psychosocial Palliative Care

Psychosocial Palliative Care

GOOD PRACTICE IN THE CARE OF THE DYING AND BEREAVED

Frances Sheldon
Macmillan Lecturer in Psychosocial Palliative Care
University of Southampton

Consultant editor: Jo Campling

Stanley Thornes (Publishers) Ltd

First published 1997 by:
Stanley Thornes (Publishers) Ltd
Ellenborough House
Wellington Street
CHELTENHAM
GL50 1YW
United Kingdom

97 98 99 00 01 / 10 9 8 7 6 5 4 3 2 1

A catalogue record for this book is available from the British Library

ISBN 0-7487-3295-0

Typeset by Florencetype Ltd, Stoodleigh, Devon
Printed and bound in Great Britain by
TJ International, Padstow, Cornwall

Dedication

To

Richard Hillier
Hazel Osborn
Keith Telford

who gave me my start in palliative care and have continued
to encourage and challenge me.

Contents

Acknowledgements   xi

Introduction   1

1 The basis of palliative care   5
  1.1 What is palliative care?   5
  1.2 Principles of palliative care   7
  1.3 Psychosocial palliative care and who delivers it   10
  1.4 Key concepts in psychosocial palliative care   10
  1.5 What the professional brings to palliative care   14

2 The cultural and spiritual context of death and bereavement   17
  2.1 Setting the scene   17
    2.1.1 The influence of culture   17
    2.1.2 Western cultural views of death   21
    2.1.3 The spiritual dimension   23
    2.1.4 Lifecourse issues   25
  2.2 Issues in practice   27
    2.2.1 Access to palliative care   27
    2.2.2 Handling conflict over cultural issues   29
    2.2.3 Spiritual care   31

**3 Social and health care policy and the development
  of palliative care**   35
  3.1 Setting the scene   35
    3.1.1 The influences on development   35
    3.1.2 The process of development   37
    3.1.3 Future trends   40
    3.1.4 The spread of palliative care   44

3.2 Issues in practice 45
    3.2.1 Over-treatment and under-treatment 45
    3.2.2 Requests for euthanasia 47
    3.2.3 Making home care possible 49

4 The individual facing death 53
4.1 Setting the scene 53
    4.1.1 Psychological responses to approaching death 53
    4.1.2 Denial 56
    4.1.3 Quality of life 57
    4.1.4 Communicating with people who are dying 58
4.2 Issues in practice 60
    4.2.1 Ethical challenges in communication 60
    4.2.2 Breaking bad news and eliciting concerns 61
    4.2.3 Working with denial 62
    4.2.4 Working with anger 65
    4.2.5 Working with depression and sadness 66
    4.2.6 Life review 67
    4.2.7 Groups for patients 69

5 Carers and families – the time before death 71
5.1 Setting the scene 71
    5.1.1 The changing nature of the family 71
    5.1.2 Conflicting demands for carers 72
    5.1.3 Support for carers 74
    5.1.4 Sexuality 75
    5.1.5 How similarly do dying people and their carers
        perceive the situation? 76
    5.1.6 The needs of children facing bereavement 77
5.2 Issues in practice 79
    5.2.1 Mapping the support networks 79
    5.2.2 The protective carer 80
    5.2.3 Meeting sexual needs 81
    5.2.4 Meeting the needs of children facing bereavement 82
    5.2.5 Family meetings 86
    5.2.6 The last days 88

6 Bereavement 90
6.1 Setting the scene 90
    6.1.1 The development of bereavement theory 91
    6.1.2 Challenges to accepted models 92
    6.1.3 New approaches to bereavement theory 95
    6.1.4 What influences the grief process? 96
    6.1.5 Pathological grief – does it exist? 98

6.1.6 Effective intervention 99
6.2 Issues in practice 100
6.2.1 Around the time of death 100
6.2.2 Assessing who is at risk in bereavement 102
6.2.3 Providing services for bereaved people 102
6.2.4 Meeting the needs of vulnerable groups 103
6.2.5 Working with difficult problems in bereavement 106

7 Working in palliative care 108
7.1 Setting the scene 108
7.1.1 Sources of stress for staff caring for people
who are dying 108
7.1.2 Teamwork in palliative care – is it effective? 112
7.1.3 Team membership 113
7.1.4 Are the dying person and their carers members
of the team? 114
7.1.5 Issues for teams 115
7.1.6 Advocacy 117
7.2 Issues in practice 117
7.2.1 Team building 117
7.2.2 Joint education 119
7.2.3 Support systems 120
7.2.4 Staff support groups 121
7.2.5 Handling conflict in teams 123

8 Living with dying 126
8.1 Preventing burnout and battle fatigue 127
8.2 The role of the arts 128
8.3 Complementary therapies 131
8.4 Assuring quality 133
8.5 Conclusion 135

References 138

Index 154

Acknowledgements

Any one who has worked for many years in a particular field will recognize my dilemma. How can I hope to identify, let alone mention, all those from whom I have learnt? Those mentioned below can only be a very few of the many to whom I owe a debt. I am most grateful to them all. Any errors and omissions are my responsibility.

Those who were dying and their carers with whom I have worked at Countess Mountbatten House, Southampton must come first. A field that I intended to stay in for just a couple of years has become a career because of what I have learnt from them about the generosity and tenacity of human beings.

Those who have been teachers and students on M.Sc. in Psychosocial Palliative Care and M.Sc. in Professional Studies at Southampton University will see how much I have learnt from them. Many of them are credited directly in the references.

The University of Southampton gave me study leave from February to September 1996, without which I could not have hoped to complete this book.

Colleagues in the Department of Social Work Studies, Southampton University covered my work while I was away. Particular thanks to Dorothy Jerome, Hazel Osborn, Sarah Munday and Bridget Wilde. Jackie Powell and Colin Pritchard have been unfailingly stimulating colleagues.

The five Macmillan Social Work Lecturers Carolyn Brodbribb, Jo Heslop, Gill Luff, David Oliviere and Ann Quinn have been a very supportive reference group. David Oliviere in particular has contributed to this book by often substituting for me and thus freeing me to write.

Past and present colleagues at Countess Mountbatten House, Southampton have since 1977 provided the environment where I learnt about excellence in palliative care. My debt to Richard Hillier is immeasurable. Sheila Lees and Graham Thorpe have set standards of integrity I have tried to follow. Pauline Turner has kept me in touch with good practice in palliative care nursing and teaching. Grateful thanks to Celia Cooke and Barbara Shaw who have continued to make me welcome in the social work team.

Marilyn Relf, Sheila Payne, Virginia Dunn and others in the Bereavement Research Forum have shown me what an interesting and complex area bereavement research is. I have valued their fellowship.

Jo Campling has acted as midwife to this book. As she has done for so many first time authors, she first made me believe I could do it, and then gave the encouragement and advice necessary to bring about its completion.

Barbara Monroe, Director of Social Work at St Christopher's Hospice is that rare being, an honest critic. If this book is helpful to practitioners much is due to her perceptive suggestions.

Keith Telford patiently tolerated my preoccupation with this book but ensured that I did not lose touch with the world outside palliative care. He has, as always, been a most significant support.

Introduction

This book is designed to help those professionals working in health and social care with the painful, challenging but often satisfying task of supporting those who are dying and those who care for them. Its focus is particularly on the psychosocial aspects of care, which may pose greater problems than the control of physical symptoms. Its main concern will be with adults who are dying and their carers. These may of course include children and the needs of children facing bereavement will certainly be considered. However, the care of dying children will not specifically be included although some of the material may have equal relevance for them. The book is directed at those who have recently qualified – whether they are nurses, social workers, therapists, doctors or clergy – who are taking responsibility for this area of care perhaps for the first time and want to offer the best possible service to their patients or clients. They may be working in specialist health services for the dying or bereaved, or they may be based in a general setting, in the community or in a hospital, where dying people form only a small proportion of their workload. Those who have been developing specialist services are building a body of knowledge and experience about what is now commonly called palliative care, and this book will draw on this. Because people who are dying require above all a holistic approach and because the psychosocial aspects of their care are not the province of any one profession, issues covered will be relevant to those working in both social and health care.

Caring for someone who is dying has always been, and continues to be, primarily carried out by families and friends. In this book they will be described by the generic term 'carer', recognizing that those carrying out this role may not always be related to the dying person, nor does the relationship always carry the positive connotations of the word 'friend'. When they have needed extra help they have called upon the resources of their community and may have found it informally in their neighbourhood or more formally in institutions with a mission to relieve distress such as hospitals or churches. However, specialist health services for the care of the dying have spread rapidly throughout the world in the last quarter of the 20th century. Since the foundation of the first modern hospice in London in 1967 such services have developed to some degree in all European countries, most comprehensively in Catalonia in Spain. Hospice care is widespread in the USA and is spreading rapidly in Asia. Australia has palliative care services well-integrated into much of its general health care provision (Hunt and McCaul, 1996). With the spread of palliative care within countries which have very varying ways of approaching death and bereavement has come a greater recognition of the need to take account of the cultural framework of people who are dying. Without this sensitive care is impossible. It has too a key influence on the ethical dilemmas which so often occur in this field. Understanding the impact of cultural issues on the care of the dying and bereaved will be an important feature of this book.

Specialist services started in the area of cancer care but it has become clear that many of the ways of working can be applied to other diseases. Many services have always been ready to support those suffering from motor neurone disease, and there has been a considerable development of services for AIDS patients. Now there is a demand that specialist services shall not be a luxury service for those 'fortunate enough' to be dying of cancer, but shall be extended to anyone at the end of their life. The issues discussed in this book will relate to people dying of any life-threatening disease, unless diseases other than cancer are specifically excluded.

Inevitably the concentration in the early days of palliative care was on developing the service. Now there is an increased interest in ensuring that professionals, whether specialist practitioners in palliative care or gener- alists, are properly prepared through education and training programmes for work in this sensitive area. Alongside this is a growing concern to understand and explore more objectively what best practice in palliative care might be, and what the experience is like for patient, carer and profes- sional. So this book draws on the growing research base in this area of care, which is struggling to find its own path and appropriate methods of enquiry (Corner, 1996). However, it also seeks to be firmly rooted in the daily experience of practice of its readers and to recognize the contribution of the reflective and experienced practitioner to theoretical development and to establishing best practice.

WHAT THIS BOOK CONTAINS

The first chapter of this book will define palliative care and identify the principles and concepts underlying it. Chapters 2–7 will be in two sections. The first section – Setting the scene – will set out current knowledge on, and attitudes to, the topic of the chapter. It will draw on recent research findings and discuss areas of debate. Without some understanding of the context in which they are working and of the current concerns of fellow professionals the new practitioner approaches each new problem with no firm basis to draw on. The references indicate where those interested can read further about the topics discussed. Building on the first section the second part of the chapter – Issues in practice – will select difficult practice issues relating to the topic of the chapter and describe current approaches and innovative ideas for improving work in these areas. Ethical and communication issues inevitably arise in relation to a particular topic and will be discussed in the chapter dealing with that topic. For those who are interested in exploring ethical or communication issues for their own sake and in more depth, Randall and Downie (1996) on palliative care ethics and Buckman (1992) on communication provide useful practical guides. While this book includes a discussion of many of the psychological therapies used in palliative care, it does not consider the full range of psychiatric interventions which may be appropriate for some dying people. Readers are advised to consult the chapter by Breitbart and Passik in the *Oxford Textbook of Palliative Medicine* for an introduction to this area of the subject (Breitbart and Passik, 1993).

Chapters 2 and 3 will look at the context for palliative care – Chapter 2 at the cultural and spiritual context of death and bereavement, and Chapter 3 at social and health care policies and the development of palliative care. In the Issues in practice section of these chapters challenges for practitioners arising from the context will be selected. In Chapter 2 these will be access to palliative care, handling conflict over cultural issues and providing spiritual care, in Chapter 3 over-treatment and under-treatment, handling requests for euthanasia and how to make care for dying people at home a possibility. Chapter 4 explores the impact of facing death on the person who is dying, and issues for staff in breaking bad news and working with powerful emotions. Chapter 5 considers the experience of the informal carers – the family and those close to the person who is dying – and issues in practice that may arise from this, including protective carers, working with children where a parent is dying and sexual needs. An analysis of current models of bereavement forms the basis of Chapter 6 with a consideration of the different types of service developed to meet identified needs. Issues in practice will look at good practice around the time of death, assessing risk in bereavement and at ways of working with particular difficulties. Chapter 7 shifts the focus and tackles working as a professional in palliative care – sources of stress, what contributes to successful interprofessional working and advocacy. The Issues in practice section concentrates on team building, managing conflict in teams and staff support. The final chapter reaffirms the link between principles and practice and considers the role of the arts in sustaining both the person who is dying and the professionals caring for them.

CONCLUSION

No book can provide an exact blueprint for what to do in any situation. Good practice in any field is constantly being reviewed. This book will have achieved its objectives if those who read it have a deeper appreciation of what the challenges are in delivering good psychosocial palliative care, understand the contributions of earlier workers and researchers in the field, and have the confidence to build on these and develop new approaches in partnership with dying people and their carers.

The basis of palliative care

1

1.1 WHAT IS PALLIATIVE CARE?

Caring for people who are dying has always been an inevitable task of professionals working in health and social care. In the last part of the 20th century this aspect of care has been particularly developed, and in 1987 palliative medicine was formally recognized by the Royal College of Physicians as a speciality within medicine in the UK. The knowledge and experience of those working with the dying and bereaved is steadily being incorporated into the training of health and social care professionals in many parts of the world. What is included in the remit of palliative care?

Definitions of palliative care have been produced by a number of organizations, e.g. the World Health Organization (1990) and the European Association for Palliative Care (1989). What they have in common is the recognition that palliative care is an active approach to the care of those whose disease is not responsive to curative treatment, and that that care should encompass physical, psychological, social and spiritual problems. Dying is considered a normal process and professionals should not seek either to hasten or to postpone death. The inclusion of psychological and social problems in the remit inevitably means that those close to the dying person are included in the care offered. The emphasis is on achieving the best possible quality of life.

There has been considerable debate about when palliative care should start. Fisher, an early pioneer, asserts that 'Palliative care is a broad band of care of indeterminate length which should start the moment the cancer is diagnosed or even before, when there is a gleam of apprehension in the patient's eye' (Fisher, 1991). However, Doyle, another much respected leader in palliative medicine, observes 'For us to propose that in the United Kingdom medical and nursing specialists in palliative care should be involved with patients from the day of diagnosis will predictably confuse patients, undoubtedly antagonise many professional colleagues, make our roles even more baffling for purchasers, and give false, totally unjustified ideas of professional grandeur' (Doyle, 1993a). Concerns at the point of diagnosis may be very different from those in the last few weeks of someone's life, even for those who are sadly found to be incurable at the time of first presenting themselves for investigation. In the early days of the hospice movement some of those involved struggled with the perception of those in generalist services and of the general public that their work was about terminal care, usually defined as the very last few days of life. The emphasis on quality of life and 'living until you die' was to counter this. Others now feel that 'palliative care' has become domi-nated by a medical approach and that 'terminal care' reflects a more holistic philosophy (Biswas, 1993).

Some confusion has also arisen from recommendations in the World Health Organization (1990) booklet, *Cancer Pain Relief and Palliative Care*, concerned particularly with improving cancer care in the developing countries. For the majority at diagnosis there is no prospect of cure, yet the lion's share of resources for cancer care is spent on the curative parts of the service. The booklet recommends much greater concentration on palliation from the start in these countries. Doyle (1993b) suggests that the extrapolation of this to the very different circumstances of the affluent west, where many more have the opportunity of curative treatment, has muddied the waters.

The National Council for Hospice and Specialist Palliative Care Services (NCHSPCS) (1995a) has distinguished between the palliative approach and specialist palliative care services. It suggests that the palliative approach is 'a vital and integral part of all clinical practice, whatever the illness or its stage' and that all professionals, whatever the setting of health care, should practise the principles of palliative care. These are described as:

- An emphasis on quality of life including good symptom control.
- Autonomy and choice.
- A holistic approach.
- The dying person and those who matter to that person as the unit of care.
- Open and sensitive communication with patients, their informal carers and professional colleagues.

Specialist palliative care services for people who are dying are based on these principles but delivered by a multiprofessional team, the majority of whose members are trained and acknowledged specialists in palliative care. Such specialist palliative care teams may be located in the commu-nity or in an acute setting, and should be available to support the patient, their informal carers and their non-specialist colleagues wherever the patient is. Increasingly they have an educational role, both in providing recognized training for palliative care specialists and more generally for other health and social care professionals, and are undertaking research. In practice specialist palliative care services tend to concentrate their efforts on those judged likely to die within 12 months, but some services may see patients at an earlier stage of their illness, perhaps only for a limited time.

1.2 PRINCIPLES OF PALLIATIVE CARE

Of course the principles of palliative care indicated above are found in many other areas of health and social care but they have particular implications in the care of the dying. A clear understanding of these principles and why they have been developed will provide a framework to support those who are trying to pick their way through the minefield of caring for people who are facing one of the most challenging and emotionally powerful crises in their life. It will become clear that how these principles are interpreted will vary to some extent with the different social and cultural backgrounds of those involved, be they patients or professionals. Many of the issues raised by putting these principles into practice will be discussed in succeeding chapters.

The ability of an individual to exercise **autonomy** and make decisions and choices about their life is much valued in the parts of Europe and the USA where palliative care first developed. The emphasis on patient autonomy and choice, in palliative care as in other fields of medicine in the latter part of the 20th century, was in part a reaction against the benevolent paternalism of doctors who had regularly kept from patients the truth about their disease because they feared the truth would be damaging to the patient (Hinton, 1967). This was particularly practised in cancer care, where palliative care first developed. During this period too a more educated population, with more opportunities for obtaining information through the media, has demanded better access to information in all areas of life and the Data Protection Act and the Patient's Charter in the UK are expressions of this. To exercise autonomy a dying person must be fully informed, or as fully informed as they wish, about what is happening to them and what the possible outcomes may be, so this principle links particularly closely to that of open communication. The choices they may want to make may be about where they die or about levels of medication, about what sort of support they want or who should know about their situation. To help them achieve what they want requires a creative and needs-led approach by professionals which does not restrict choices to the services that are currently available, or to standard ways of doing things. Mesler has shown in his sensitive qualitative study of hospices in the north-eastern USA how the constraints of controlling symptoms, the state of the disease, whether the patient is at home or an in-patient and the limits set on their own involvement by staff may all circumscribe the autonomy of the patient even when staff have it as a key objective (Mesler, 1994–95).

Naturally respect for the principle of autonomy implies respect both for the autonomy of those close to the patient and for the autonomy of the professionals involved in the care, as well as for that of the patient. Professionals cannot be required to act in a way which they consider infringes their own autonomy. This is particularly relevant to the question of euthanasia.

The understanding of what patient autonomy may mean has become more complex as palliative care is offered to those from ethnic minorities in the UK and as it has developed beyond its Northern European and North American base. The different weight given to the opinion of senior or male members of the family which may form part of the culture of some Asian or Arab societies needs to be taken into account. Patients should not be forced to be autonomous where they do not wish to be, either in the UK or in Singapore, but sensitive enquiry is required too, in case the crisis of facing their own death is bringing about change in long-held beliefs and practices and a wish for greater self-determination. Clarke and her colleagues (Clarke, Finlay and Campbell, 1991) have shown how challenging it may be for staff working with a patient from another culture where views about patient autonomy are different.

It has become clear that many dying people, perhaps the majority, value **open and sensitive communication** about the issues facing them. Hinton (1967) was one of the first to show that discussion of the outcome of an incurable disease with patients may be welcomed, and may be preferable to the isolation, suspicion and uncertainty which they may experience if the truth is kept from them. Professionals involved in such communication must understand the despair and fear which the prospect of death may evoke, and tailor that communication to the pace of the patient. Similar understanding of the power of standing close to death is required in dealing with relatives and friends of the patient, and with other professionals working alongside whose less frequent exposure to death may make it more frightening to them than to those who meet it every day.

When it is clear that life will end in the near future the quality of the life that is left becomes a central concern for the person who is dying and those around him or her. Only the person who is dying can define what **quality of life** means to them. Certainly there are common ideas in every society about what is a good life or a good death, and it is impossible for those living in a particular society not to be influenced by the views of that society about this. However, it is very important for those working with the dying to try to understand what quality of life means for this individual dying person. One may find it in enjoying nature, another in having more possessions than a neighbour, another in relationships with friends and family. For one homeless dying man quality of life was returning to camp in a particular bus shelter. Because the needs and wishes of patients and their carers may change, and change fast as the disease progresses, a continual review of the goals for care is required to keep pace. Good palliative care demands a dynamic approach to care.

A holistic approach involves valuing all the characteristics and past experience of this person, not just seeing them in terms of their diagnosis or presenting problem. It is the care of the mind and spirit as well as of the body. Dame Cicely Saunders, the founder of the modern hospice movement in the UK, coined the term 'total pain' to encompass the range of physical, emotional, social and spiritual difficulties which may face the dying person (Saunders, 1993). It is becoming clearer that while control of physical pain usually comes top of the list of concerns for those who are dying, it is very closely followed by concerns about family and dependence (Rathbone *et al.*, 1994; Heaven and Maguire, 1995). Achieving a holistic approach to care is likely to require the skills and experience of several members of the professional team, but it also needs each individual member of that team to take account of areas which may not be their primary concern – the doctor of the relationships within the family, the social worker of the significance of regular medication, the nurse of the questioning of long-held religious belief. Clearly each member of the team cannot be equally skilled in all areas, but each must recognize the importance of all parts of the picture, and value and respect the knowledge and skills others contribute. Such an approach also demands a personal and human contact with the dying person which yet retains the professional distance necessary to continuing to work in close contact with emotional pain and despair.

A holistic view necessarily takes into account the relationships of the dying person, but palliative care has gone further than many other areas of health care in asserting that **the patient and those who matter to the patient form the unit of care**. This is based on a systemic view of relationships which recognizes that each individual affects, and is affected by, those closest to them. This does not mean that the views of relatives will be weighed more heavily those of the dying person, but that the interdependence of all parties is understood. The pain of the family is different but may be as great, sometimes greater than that of the dying person. Making this a principle of palliative care creates ethical challenges, and requires careful balancing of the possibly conflicting views and needs of patient and carer. A non-judgemental approach to the wide variety of ways in which families and friends may relate to each other is essential here.

1.3 PSYCHOSOCIAL PALLIATIVE CARE AND WHO DELIVERS IT

This book focuses on the psychosocial elements of palliative care. These are the psychological experience of facing death for the dying person and the impact on those close to them, which links closely to the spiritual framework of those concerned, and the social factors that influence the experience. In addition the experience for those working or acting as volunteers with people who are dying and bereaved has always been a concern in palliative care. So a consideration of what helps or hinders staff and volunteers in working in this area of care must form part of the remit too. However, acceptance of the concept of 'total pain' means that taking account of the influence of each element of this – physical, psychological, social, spiritual – on the other and on the whole must be part of the approach to care. So a book on the psychosocial aspects of palliative care must also be concerned with how physical symptoms interact with these. The patient's anxieties about who will look after their children when they are dead, even about how to pay the gas bill now, have an impact on their experience of pain, and their understanding of what the whole experience of illness means certainly will (Barkwell, 1991). Leriche's (1939) dictum 'Pain is the result of a conflict between a stimulus and the whole individual' is extended by Bendelow and Williams (1995) 'Rather than reducing pain to a mere physiological "symptom", it must be seen as physical and emotional, biological and cultural, even spiritual and existential'. Equally, persistent vomiting or diarrhoea may well affect a patient's view of their God and their relationship with their partner. For this reason the psychosocial aspects of palliative care have to be the concern of all members of the professional team. This is the implication of the principle of the holistic approach. Different professionals in the team can be expected to have different degrees of knowledge and skill in this area, and some of that will depend on the setting in which they work. Specialist palliative care nurses working in the community have more opportunity to develop a deeper understanding of the variety of ways families deal with illness than ward-based nurses who may have only brief contacts with a family over a couple of days of an admission. Social workers and clinical psychologists will, by virtue of the emphasis in their training on the psychosocial areas, have a head start over the doctor who covers these alongside the vast area of physical medicine.

1.4 KEY CONCEPTS IN PSYCHOSOCIAL PALLIATIVE CARE

In addition to the principles underlying palliative care discussed earlier, a number of concepts have been influential in the development of this field and an understanding of them will strengthen the practice of any professional. These are:

- Attachment.
- Loss.
- Meaning.
- Equity.

Bowlby (1969) developed a body of theory around the concept of **attachment** from his studies of young children's relationships with their mothers. Key points are that the child will feel secure in the presence of someone stronger and wiser (most frequently their mother) to whom they are attached, will seek that person if sensing a threat, and will protest and experience distress if they cannot have access to that person. There are inevitably some cultural differences in the styles of attachment that children develop but the phenomenon has been found across a number of cultures (Parkes, Stevenson-Hinde and Marris, 1991). Colin Murray Parkes built on this theory in developing his model of adult bereavement (Parkes, 1986) and Robert Weiss (1991) proposes that the attachment relationships of adults will be similar to those of children except that the relationship is more likely to be between two equals, to have a sexual element and to be able to be sustained without such discomfort during periods of physical separation. Parkes and Weiss would agree that if there is a threat to the continuation of the relationship the attached adult will experience a sense of apprehension, even fear, a compulsion to search for that person and difficulty in attending to other areas of life. When some one is known to have a life-threatening illness these emotions are triggered for those who are attached to them, as indeed they may be for the dying person themselves in relation to their attachments, as they become aware of their situation. Once the death has actually occurred the survivor's grief will, at least initially, very frequently contain these elements.

The experience of **loss**, or rather of a series of losses, is indissolubly part of the experience of dying and of bereavement. As the disease takes hold the sick person will have to face changes in physical functioning which may limit the possibility of continuing to work, affect close relationships or force a change of home. The person who is bereaved faces a loss of their role in relation to that person – parent, child, partner – and the end of a unique relationship. Parkes (1971) has suggested that each of us develop an 'assumptive world' which is made up of our perceptions of past experience, and our expectations of, and plans for the future. Major changes which are lasting take place over a short time, giving little time for preparation, and affect large areas of our assumptive world he calls psychosocial transitions. These are likely to be resisted, to be painful and lonely, and the loss of such a large part of the assumptive world may make the areas that remain seem threatened. A young woman whose much loved mother had died 10 days after the birth of her first child began to find herself becoming very anxious if her young, fit husband was at all late coming home from work. She could no longer take for granted that he was safe if she could not see him.

How individuals deal with the losses involved in facing their own death, or the death of someone they are close to, will be affected by how the society that they live in responds to this event. Western society in the late 20th century has often been characterized, rather simplistically, as a 'death-denying' society. This view is now being challenged and a more discriminating understanding of this complex area is emerging (Walter, 1994). This will be explored in more depth in Chapter 2. The coping strategies that an individual has learnt through their experience of earlier crises may well be those that they bring into play now, but it is most important that professionals working with those who are dying recognize that this time has the potential to be a time of growth and development, when new strategies are chosen. A man who had been a senior manager in a public service organization and whose professional and personal life had been characterized by a driving energy and determination to succeed, faced his death with a calm, contemplative acceptance which surprised and even disconcerted his family, who expected him to fight against the disease until the last minute. Chapter 4 will consider these issues further.

Of course many losses may bring with them some element of gain. Some people who are dying record how much they have valued the increased closeness with their family that the experience has brought. Bereaved people may in time reflect how they have gained in self-reliance. However, professionals in palliative care are likely to be working with people at times when it is the negative aspect of the change that is predominantly felt.

However, it is not the fact of the loss but the **meaning** of the loss for each individual that gives it its unique power. The meaning of the death of a wife may for one man be that the world is an entirely arbitrary place where fairness is not to be expected, for another that the natural end of her life has come. Each of us builds up over time a personal meaning system defined by Dittman-Kohli (1990) as 'the pattern of valuations and concepts by which individuals represent to themselves at a given phase of existence what they believe and want in relation to their own life and self'. This personal system of meaning may derive from such sources as personal relationships, spiritual experience, creativity, hedonism or the wish to leave a legacy. Cultural factors and position in the lifespan will also influence it. Frankl, a Jewish psychotherapist, drawing on his experience as a prisoner in a concentration camp in the Second World War (1987), suggests there is an ultimate meaning and purpose in the world for each of us to discover, and that each of us searches for a meaning specific to the particular situation we are in. Through taking responsibility for our attitude to that situation, we may develop a meaning that makes it possible to control our view of the situation, even if it is not possible to control the situation itself. In his position, which he characterized as 'a provisional existence of unknown limit', his continued living subject to the arbitrary whim of the camp guards, he found meaning in the remembrance of the love of his wife and in a vision of himself lecturing on his experience at sometime in the future. Frankl's insights have relevance for those facing that 'provisional existence of unknown limit' which the diagnosis of a terminal illness brings, and for professionals involved in their care. Hearing the anguished 'why' questions of the dying and bereaved, encouraging them to explore ideas about the possible answers without offering any, gives them an opportunity to find their own meaning. A note of caution here. Meaning may change over time with further reflection. One bereaved man observed of the failure of others to offer him the warmth he was desperate for 'I used to think people were wicked but it's not so, they are just busy, busy, busy' (*The Life That's Left*, CTVC, 1977). Meanings will not necessarily be positive. Barkwell (1991) studied a group of 100 cancer patients at the terminal stage of the disease. She found that they were for the most part divided between those who saw their illness as a challenge, as a punishment or as an enemy. Those who saw their illness as a punishment experienced more pain and depression than those who understood it as a challenge. Wortman and Silver (1989) have pointed out that those who have experienced the death of a child can very seldom give it a positive meaning in western societies in the 20th century, whereas parents in the past have, at least publicly, been able to see it in terms of a happy life for the child in heaven (T.R.S., 1856).

The concept of **equity** has had an interesting history in palliative care. Part of the initial impetus for the development of the hospice movement was the recognition that dying patients were not receiving as good a service as those for whom there was some hope of cure. Saunders' awareness of the unrelieved pain and isolation of these patients impelled her to go to train as a doctor on her path to founding St Christopher's Hospice (Saunders, 1993). Then hospices developed in the UK in response to local, often voluntary, initiatives, seldom following any assessment of whether the need for specialist care was greater in that geographical area than in a neighbouring district, and they developed largely in the area of cancer care. This produced impassioned criticism from some quarters. 'Why should only the minority who die of malignancies – and precious few of them – be singled out for *de luxe* dying? And why should a large and general need be left to the scanty and scandalously choosy efforts of a patchwork of local charities with one hand in the coffers of the NHS and the other in the church bazaar economy?' (Douglas, 1991). A survey by the NCHSPCs (1995b) found that people from black and ethnic minorities in England were not achieving equal access to specialist palliative care with the white majority population. The elderly are thought by some to have been neglected in favour of younger people who are dying or bereaved (Cohen, 1996). Certainly specialist palliative care services in the UK were generally slow to recognize the needs of residents of nursing homes for palliative care and these residents are predominantly elderly. Those aged over 80 dying in South Australia are much less likely to be involved with a hospice than those under 40 (Hunt and McCaul, 1996). Now Health Authorities are required to purchase appropriate palliative care for all their residents and a more equitable spread of services may be achieved in Britain. Where palliative care is developing in other countries the equitable impulse to improve the care of dying patients finds similarly uneven expression in the establishment of new services. Only in the province of Catalonia in Spain has the coverage been more universal from an early date (Gomez-Batiste *et al.*, 1992). Equity is of course not just about treating equal things equally, but also about treating unequal things unequally. Ignatieff (1990) observes 'There is also a contradiction in the heart of the Welfare State, between the respect we owe persons as individuals and as fellow human beings. The first type of respect requires us to treat them differently, unequally; the second to treat them like every other human being. In the Welfare State individuals are supposed to be treated equally, as if their needs were all the same. Yet our needs are not the same. What means respect to you may not be what respect means to me'. The ethical dilemmas that this can pose in palliative care will be examined in Chapter 2.

1.5 WHAT THE PROFESSIONAL BRINGS TO PALLIATIVE CARE

No less than the dying person and their carers the professionals or volunteers in this field bring with them their own views about death and bereavement which may derive from past experience either in their personal lives or at work. Some of the influences on them they may share with their patients or clients. For those living in Western societies death from disease at a young age is unusual, almost regarded as an affront. Accidents have overtaken the cancers as the greatest cause of death for those under 15 in the UK. Life expectancy is still increasing. Death comes in late-middle age or in old age, often following a period of degenerative disease. The death of a young person may therefore be particularly challenging to professionals. Many of the pioneers in palliative care were driven by their experience at work, usually in hospital, of people who were dying being neglected and shunned by doctors and nurses more interested in those who had some hope of cure. Mills, Davis and Macrae (1994) give a graphic picture of the sort of care that they were reacting against – the pleas of patients too weak to feed themselves being ignored, patients dying alone and untended. Such motivation may be found less frequently now that palliative care has become more routinized (James and Field, 1992) and incorporated into mainstream services. Some have always been motivated by personal experience of the death of someone close to them and it continues to be a powerful factor in inducing some to become a volunteer in a hospice. Religious faith drew many in the early days, as the number of hospices called after saints testifies. These influences from culture and experience will inevitably shape the attitudes of professionals in this field and provide a base from which they develop their own individual system of meaning.

However, there are some particular values too which are implicit in the principles of palliative care. A respect for the right of the patient to be self-determining within the confines set by the rights of others, and a determination to empower them to be so, is one. Allied to this is a non-judgemental approach valuing the uniqueness of this individual. This does not mean endorsing everything that they do or have done. Staff at a hospice caring for a dying man admitted from prison where he had been serving a life sentence for murdering a child could not avoid making a judgement about that, but had to offer him the same level of sensitive care that was being offered to the good citizen in the next bed. As Stedeford (1984) observes 'How a person dies depends on at least three factors: the way he has lived, the type of illness, and the quality of care. Staff share grief about the first and second, but only the third is their responsibility'. Maintaining such a non-judgemental stance may require considerable discussion and sharing of frustrations within the team in rela-tion to particular patients or carers.

The qualities of empathy and genuineness are central to palliative care, as they are to many areas of health and social care. Listening to the pain of those who are dying, particularly their despair as they face leaving those they love and with aims unfulfilled, can be very testing for those who hear this day after day (Lanceley, 1995). Two attributes that help here are the ability to balance the reality of the imminence of death with the hope of achieving some continuing small pleasures in life with patient and carers, and an unsentimental belief in the potential for change and development within every human being even in the worst crisis. Self-awareness and taking responsibility for one's own actions and feelings in the professional role are a further safeguard against over-involvement and emotional exhaustion on the one hand and a distanced remoteness on the other. Chapters 7 and 8 will look at the ways that staff support and develop-ment can help professionals in palliative care to maintain all these difficult balances.

1.6 CONCLUSION

This chapter has set out the remit of palliative care and has described the principles underpinning practice for anyone working in palliative care. It forms the backcloth against which all the issues dealt with in subsequent chapters must be considered. The next step is to examine the cultural and spiritual context of death and bereavement which will inform both the individual's experience, and the way that a particular society organizes services to deal with that experience.

The cultural and spiritual context of death and bereavement

2.1 SETTING THE SCENE

2.1.1 The influence of culture

Every culture develops particular ways of handling the key life-cycle events such as birth and death, and even those who see themselves as having rejected much of their cultural heritage may turn to those familiar paths at such times. English couples who have no religious belief often seek a marriage ceremony in a church. Culture is 'a set of guidelines (both explicit and implicit) which individuals inherit as members of a particular society, and which tells them how to view the world, how to experience it emotionally, and how to behave in it in relation to other people, to supernatural forces or gods, and to the natural environment. It also provides them with a way of transmitting these guidelines to the next generation – by the use of symbols, language, art and ritual' (Helman, 1994). As Mead observes, it includes both the over-arching institutions of society and 'the small intimate habits of daily life, such as preparing or eating food, or hushing a child to sleep', and all is part of an interlinked whole (Mead, 1953). One particular piece of behaviour such as a mourning ritual cannot be detached but must be seen for how it fits into the larger pattern.

Helman's definition is clearly not just about people with non-white skins, although the term 'culturally sensitive practice' is often still used in the UK to refer to work only with those from black or ethnic minority populations. This ignores the fact that many black people may be the third or fourth generation of their family to live in the UK and may have fully taken on the culture of the majority white population. It also disregards the different cultural background that may be shared by some people with white skins, e.g. those with an Irish cultural heritage or the regional variations even in such a small country as the UK. Clearly the restriction of the term has grown up because of the recognition that, as we shall see later in the chapter, the services provided for minority groups have often disregarded their particular needs. However, in reality we all have a culture which may feel comfortable and right for us, but is not therefore necessarily superior to any other. Culture may have a close link to a religion. Most importantly it is dynamic. It is constantly changing in response to economic and environmental factors acting on those individuals who subscribe to it.

Clark (1982) has described the changes in the cultural practices around death in the Yorkshire village of Staithes between the early and later years of the 20th century. The professionalization of death by the end of the century meant that the roles of the group of women who were recognized as 'qualified' to lay out a corpse and of the village joiner in making the coffin had been superseded by the funeral director, to some degree because death now more often took place in a more distant hospital rather than at home, which in itself was a response to the changes in medical practice. These changes mirrored those going on in other parts of the UK. In one particular, Staithes had not followed the rest of the country – in retaining a preference for burial over cremation. Clark speculates that this was due to a deep-seated preference arising from the earlier cultural norm and based on respect for the worth of a person who has died, rather than because the crematorium was some distance away, potentially increasing the cost and trouble of the funeral. This detailed analysis of change in one small village reminds us of the need to understand very local issues as well as those stemming from the broader religious or national factors which make up the cultural 'baggage' of the individual before us.

One situation where the dynamic of change is most obvious is among those who migrate to an area where the culture is different from their own. Such individuals may well take on many of the behaviours and ways of thinking of that culture. In time minority groups develop the same disease patterns as the host culture. For their children, born and growing up in a different culture and country from their parents, there is the challenge of deciding what elements from each culture to adopt for themselves and how to deal with any conflict that these choices may create with their family of origin. Peoples have always moved and mixed but today have the potential to move further and faster than ever before. To some degree this has brought a greater respect for other cultures, but whatever the spectrum of feeling about those different from ourselves in a particular society, health and social care systems are in many countries expected at the very least to pay lip service to providing equal levels of service for

citizens. This will certainly involve having access to good general information about different cultures. Neuberger's book *Caring for Dying
People of Different Faiths* (1987) provides a good detailed guide in the
palliative care field to the beliefs, customs and rituals of the major faiths.
As she is constantly at pains to point out, this knowledge is not necessarily a guide to how the man or woman in front of you will behave or
think. Each person will make up their own individual mix which may
depend on whether they prefer the liberal or traditional wing of their
group, whether their community is a significant minority within a host
country or numbered in ones and twos, the laws of the country and their
own life experience.

What are the areas that require particular sensitivity when someone is
dying – whatever culture they come from? Attitudes to illness, life and
death are all culturally determined. The view that sickness is a punishment and that long life is a sign of virtue are all found to varying extents
in Christianity, Islam, Judaism and Hinduism. Buddhists may refuse pain
relief because they fear their perceptions may be blunted, hampering their
search for the heightened awareness that is to bring freedom and peace
(Neuberger, 1993). What is identified as a symptom and how it is described
is culturally determined (Macleod, 1996). The word 'sore' in the question
'Is it sore?' has a slightly different meaning in the north-east of England
from in the south. The approach to the possibility of death may vary
considerably, from the more fatalistic view in Islam though this is not
universal even for those of this faith (Sheldon, 1995), to the importance
of preserving hope in the Jewish faith, which may sometimes lead to a
wish to preserve life at all cost (Abeles, 1991). There may be very real
conflicts working with Jewish patients when the professional wishes to
adhere to the palliative care principle, outlined in Chapter 1, of open
communication about the outcome of the disease and to cease curative
treatment. The resolution lies in respecting the right of the patient not to
know what is happening, but also the right of the professional not to give
treatment which they do not consider effective (Randall and Downie,
1995) – and the sensitive communication of this.

Views of the body are another key area. Modesty is very important
particularly for women in Arab cultures, and to bare an arm for a drip
may be unthinkable for strict Muslim women when a man is present. Even
in the UK with its less strict cultural approach to modesty, the widespread
dislike of mixed wards in hospitals has reversed a trend of the 1980s when
it was sought to introduce them on economic grounds. For Sikhs the
importance of wearing one of the five symbols of their religion, the kaccha
(underpants), at all times is a religious duty. For them too hair loss is
particularly distressing as the kesh, the uncut hair worn in a bun, is another
of these symbols. For women with breast cancer having chemotherapy in
the USA studied by Freedman (1994), hair loss was the most distressing

aspect of their situation, but for a different reason. The value that their culture sets on personal appearance, the hair as part of this and the visibility of the loss to the women meant that it brought home to them, more sharply than even the loss of their breast which was easier to conceal from themselves and others, what was happening to them.

Food is another source of cultural difference. Each culture has a range of prohibitions for particular foods which may have a religious base, like the prohibition on eating pork for Muslims, or may derive from other values. The British refusal to eat horse is a source of surprise to their neighbours in Belgium and stems from a particular value ascribed to domesticated animals. Not only the food itself but the way it is prepared may be an issue for the stricter adherents of a faith. Both strict Jews and strict Muslims entering hospital might wish to have food brought in or eat from disposable plates. Where fasting is part of a religious tradition this may have a major impact on the effect of drugs when someone is dying. Ways of serving and eating food are all influenced by cultural patterns. Where there are rules stemming from religion behind these differences, failure to observe them may be believed to have a particularly powerful and damaging effect on the present state or afterlife of the person who is dying.

Finally the role of the family and individual family members may be seen very differently. Uncles or cousins may be ascribed a much greater importance in a Hindu society than they are in the UK. In general there are often considerable differences around the role and status of women. Baider and De-Nour's (1987) research on Arab women in Israel with breast cancer showed that their source of support, their confidante, was much more likely to be their mother or sister than their husband. The study by the National Council for Hospice and Specialist Care (NCHSPCS, 1995b) of palliative care services for people from black and ethnic minorities in the UK singled out the difficulties particularly for Asian women, both in making their needs known and in securing practical help from men in the family when they were ill. Oliviere (1993) cautions against bringing Western values to cultures where women's main roles are still seen as motherhood and homemaking. Handling conflicts over cultural issues will be considered in the Issues in practice section.

Many of the rituals around death and bereavement may have to be performed by particular family members and considerable guilt may arise if this is not possible (Firth, 1993). In the UK the expectation that the eldest son will automatically take responsibility for arranging a funeral for an elderly widowed parent is disappearing but many families feel the need to explain to hospital staff why it is more convenient for someone else to do it, in deference to the old almost forgotten custom. There will be further discussion of cultural issues in relation to bereavement in Chapter 6.

2.1.2 Western cultural views of death

There has been a long-running debate about the extent to which in Northern Europe and the USA contemporary society is death denying and treats death as a taboo topic. Those who assert that it is take their cue from Gorer (1965) and Aries (1974). The first writing in the UK, the second taking a more European canvas, both lament what they see as the decline of rituals around death and bereavement in the 20th century and fear for the psychological health of the bereaved. Gorer uses his famous phrase 'the pornography of death' to explain the seeming inconsistency of a society where it seems unacceptable for bereaved people to express their feelings, but yet there is a flood of newspaper articles and television programmes about violent death and serious illness. Aries does take rather a simplistic view of approaches to death in earlier ages, where the accounts we have may be as much of what people at the time wished to believe happened as of reality. The solemn deathbed scene at home was always more likely to be available to the rich than the poor. The ritual periods for wearing black or reducing social contact could become a straitjacket rather than a support for some bereaved people. However, it is true that, like the people of Staithes, the majority of people in Europe and the USA in the second half of the 20th century are dying in the antiseptic atmosphere of the hospital where professionals manage the environment. With the decline in church membership the church is no longer central to the process of death, merely for many offering an acceptable way of enabling the disposal of the body.

On the other side, sociologists like Armstrong (1987) have argued that, with the legal requirement to register deaths and the medicalization of death and bereavement, death had actually become much more public. Blauner (1966) asserted that death is not taboo but hidden. His contention is that death now commonly occurs in old age rather than at any age as in the past and the elderly in Western society are not central to the operation of that society. They do not leave the same sort of gap as the death of a younger, economically active person. Walter in his sociological critique of attitudes to and behaviour around death and bereavement has argued for a more discriminating approach which recognizes the complexity of the situation (1994).

He suggests that in Western society there have been three cultural approaches to death, each with particular features which he discusses in detail. His overall framework is as shown in Figure 2.1

Traditional death is the system whose demise is mourned by Gorer and Aries. Modern death, with the expert doctors who control death and tell you how to mourn, has hidden death in hospitals and in old age. Neo-modern death he characterizes as 'the revival of death'. There is an increased interest in the ways other cultures manage death, particularly

	Traditional	Modern	Neo-modern
Bodily context	Death quick and frequent	Death hidden	Death prolonged
Social context	Community	Public versus private	Private becomes public
Authority	Religion	Medicine	Self

Figure 2.1 Cultural responses to death. Redrawn with permission from Walter, T. (1994) *The Revival of Death*, Routledge. London.

cultures seen as more simple and direct, although as Walter points out there is rather a selective interest here and seldom a rejection of modern medical treatment. Alongside this there is a particular value set on expressing emotion, which is discouraged or encouraged in prescribed ways only in modern death. A central theme is that the individual dying or bereaved person chooses their own way to respond to their situation and should not have to fit into one culturally prescribed way. The neo-modern approach draws on elements of both the other approaches but without acknowledging the contradictions which may arise when the roots of each are so different. Walter's aim in delineating these three systems is to 'illuminate the varied and often conflicting elements that make up the death culture of today'. Different generations, different members of the same family, men or women may feel more comfortable with one approach rather than another and this can produce considerable tensions at a time of heightened emotion when someone is dying.

Professionals in specialist palliative care tended in the early days of its development to subscribe to the modern death approach, and often promoted a particular way of facing death and bereavement. As we shall see later on, the way that the writings of key figures like Elisabeth Kuebler-Ross and Colin Murray Parkes have been used to write prescriptions for how to die and how to grieve have been part of this. Now the neo-modern view is becoming more prevalent, indeed the principles of autonomy, open communication and respecting the individual's own view of quality of life, identified as core principles in Chapter 1, are basic to that approach. Only one thing is certain – that the ideas current about how to handle death and bereavement will continue to develop and change in response to the other changes in a particular society. What is important is that professionals working with vulnerable people understand where the variety of approaches spring from and do not seek to impose their own idea of what is 'the proper way' to die or to grieve, but are ready to engage in discussion about these issues with individuals and families who wish it. This stance is clearly influenced by the ideas Walter characterizes as neo-modern. To maintain this receptiveness and openness requires the self-awareness and self-monitoring described in Chapter 1, and also a working environment that promotes it. The characteristics of this will be discussed in Chapter 7.

2.1.3 The spiritual dimension

In virtually everything that is written on the spiritual dimension in palliative care the authors are careful to remind us that spiritual is not the same as 'religious'. This relates both to a relatively recent broadening of view about this (Speck, 1993) and to the continuing difficulty professionals find in tackling this area. If 'spiritual' means 'religious faith and affiliation' it can all be left to the chaplain – so the defence runs. If it has a broader meaning then each member of the team will need to consider their responsibilities in this area. Who may offer spiritual care and the issues involved will be explored in the Issues in practice section.

So what does the spiritual dimension cover? Lunn (1993) suggests it is the essence of what it means to be human, ultimate concerns – questions about meaning and values – and our deepest relationships, whether with others, with God or gods, or with ourselves. Religion he describes as 'the corporate, organized and outward expression of belief systems and an attempt to describe and express faith, ordinarily in community'. King and colleagues (1994) add to our understanding by separating out the philosophical from the spiritual. They use the word 'spiritual' to indicate an individual's belief in a power outside of themselves and their own existence (separate from the concept that they have about that power), whereas they use the term 'philosophical' to describe a search for existential meaning in a particular life situation where there is no belief in or recourse to a power outside themselves. Studies have shown (Seale and Cartwright, 1994) that while formal religious affiliation is declining in the UK, a large proportion of the population still have spiritual beliefs as defined by King and his fellow researchers.

There have been some attempts to examine the effect of spiritual factors on the course and outcome of illness. However, as King and his colleagues point out, there are considerable difficulties about measuring the strength and influence of a belief system. Use of religious activity such as membership of a church as a proxy measure is of limited value as it is too blunt to distinguish even between those with a religious faith and is of no help with those with other spiritual or philosophical approaches. Paloutzian and Ellison's Spiritual Well-Being Scale (Ellison, 1982) is an attempt to distinguish between these different elements but doubt has been cast on its validity and reliability. Using a combination of semi-structured interview, the General Household questionnaire and a Beliefs questionnaire developed for the research, King and colleagues studied 300 in-patients admitted consecutively to an acute hospital at admission and 6 months later. They found that only 26 did not admit to religious or spiritual beliefs or a philosophy of life and that those who expressed lower strength of belief had a significantly better clinical outcome at 6 months than those expressing an average or higher strength of belief. The explanation for this latter finding could relate to a greater interest in spiritual issues by those with poorer prognosis or less fear of death by those with a strong faith and therefore less struggle for survival. Seale and Cartwright (1994) found in their national survey of a sample of deaths in 1987 that those said by relatives to have a strong religious faith were also said to be more accepting of death than those with less conviction. This could, of course, be because those relatives wished to believe this. Research in this area is at an early stage but it does reinforce the case for recognizing the importance of spiritual factors alongside the psychosocial and physical when considering 'total pain'.

One aspect of the spiritual dimension in palliative care that has had some attention from researchers is that of hope. A review of the literature on hope by McGee (1984) indicates that hope is widely agreed as having four main elements: it is concerned with the future, motivating, action orientated and involves expectancy. It may be influenced by internal factors such as the personality and coping mechanisms of the individual which have in turn been developed as a result of life experiences. Seligman's identification of 'learned helplessness' is relevant here (Seligman, 1975). He suggests that some individuals learn that life will be a succession of problems, that these problems will cast a shadow over their whole life and that they are to some degree responsible for creating them, whereas others learn that each crisis is a one-off event for which others are responsible and that it will not necessarily affect the whole of their life. The former group are more likely to experience depressive illness and to be overwhelmed by life events, whereas the latter group may more easily maintain hope. Current energy levels may also be a factor but Herth (1990) has shown that this is not necessarily so with people who are dying, although for them the energy required to deal with uncontrolled pain may overwhelm them. External factors that influence hope are the culture in which the person lives and their current environment, which included both the physical setting and the relationships that are possible with carers and others. High levels of hope have been found to be linked with high levels of coping (Herth, 1989).

Herth's research (1989, 1990), which includes people with life-threatening illness, is particularly relevant to practitioners in palliative care. In one study (Herth, 1990), she carried out a series of three interviews with 10 adults who were aware that they were terminally ill and given a prognosis of less than 6 months. She identified a number of strategies used by these patients to foster hope and other factors which hindered it. These will be discussed in the section on Issues in practice later in this chapter. Much of the still limited research in this area has been carried out with cancer patients who are white Europeans or North Americans, so cannot be assumed to apply to those from other cultures or with other diseases. Qualitative studies like Herth's provide ideas for others to take further.

There are still issues to be teased out around the inter-related areas of hope, coping and denial. A number of studies are concerned about unrealistic hope (McGee, 1984) and see one of the professional roles as keeping hope realistic. Van der Niet's study (1995) of specialist palliative care nurses' perceptions of hope and of their role in maintaining it for patients found this was a preoccupation for most of her respondents. The difficulty here is drawing the line between realistic and unrealistic hope, and who should do it. Professional and patient may be drawing on different values and areas of knowledge in making such an assessment. Professionals, even palliative care specialists, are still rather poor at forecasting life expectancy and the actual course of this person's illness (Robbins *et al.*, 1995). When unrealistic hope shades into denial is a judgement that is virtually impossible to make. The autonomous patient has the responsibility for their own actions and beliefs, provided the professional has done all that is reasonable to inform them (Randall and Downie, 1995). What is practically more important is the effect that unrealistic hope or denial may have on those dependent on the patient. This will be explored in Chapter 4.

2.1.4 Lifecourse issues

A more subtle approach is developing in palliative care to understanding the impact of dying at different points in the life span both on that person themselves and on those around them. Seale (1991) has shown that the characteristics of those dying from cancer and those dying from other causes are different in important respects. Cancer patients are more likely to die at a younger age, to have a shorter but more intense illness requiring more admissions, to have more relatives able to look after them and who agreed that the death had come at the right time (both because the relatives are likely to be younger as well and because they do not become exhausted by a long illness). Hospice and palliative care is most developed in the field of cancer care, so staff are more likely to be dealing with patients with these characteristics, and the style and principles of care may be more suited to this group than to older patients with other diseases. Certainly there is a debate about whether older people who grew up in an age where the doctor was given a more powerful status really wish to be partners in their care and subscribe so fully to the principles of autonomy and open communication as younger people may.

Older people may have rather different attitudes to death. Munnichs (1987) distinguished between attitudes to finitude, i.e. the understanding that my life will have an inevitable end, and attitudes to death and dying when it is actually faced. His research with people who were elderly in the Netherlands showed that as they became older they increasingly accepted the inevitability of death. From his studies of elderly people facing relocation in the USA, Tobin (1991) concluded that it is when individuals perceive that they are 'old' that they accept that death is near, and they become more concerned with the actual process of dying and not losing control (but autonomy is particularly valued in American society). He suggested that religion may offer a type of magical coping to those with a faith facing death – but again this is a society where religion and religious observance has a more significant place than it does, for example, in the UK. He emphasizes particularly the importance of maintaining 'personhood', a sense of self and of meaning in life for people in advanced old age.

Younger people, whether they are family carers or professionals, who have not yet made these adjustments to the inevitability of death may find the calm acceptance of some elderly people quite challenging, especially if they have been led to believe that anger is an inevitable response to losing one's own life. On the other hand it is important not to assume that just because someone is old in years that they have accepted that they are 'old'. One active 82-year-old was furious at the possibility of being cut off in her prime – all her siblings had lived until well into their 90s. Making individualized care a reality is the only answer here. Only further research will reveal whether the greater acceptance of death in many elderly people is a cohort effect, i.e. appearing in today's elderly people because of their particular set of life experiences, or whether it is an element of growing old for any elderly person.

Since death at a young age is now unexpected in western societies, the death of a young person tends to create more anger and more questions about why this is happening. These relate not just to the quest for explanations of the reasons for physical disease, but to how this unexpected event can be fitted into the questioner's general understanding of how the world works and notions of fairness. 'Untimely death' is a concept which only has meaning within the expectation that there is an accepted lifespan (perhaps threescore years and 10), but is one that has particular relevance for the parents or grandparents of a young person who is dying and Parkes (1975) has shown that young widows and widowers experiencing untimely (and sudden) death are more likely to have a difficult bereavement. Walter (1994) charts how social attitudes to child death have changed by quoting advice from *The Lady* magazine in 1899 that a woman should mourn a grandparent for nine months but a child only for three months.

As already indicated in Chapter 1, if a professional is a member of a society where these attitudes are current they may well find dealing with a younger patient particularly testing. The result can be a greater level of personal involvement in such situations. The professional, or their children, may be of a similar age. This may lead to difficulty in maintaining that more objective and professional stance, a protection for both the professional and the dying person. Another effect can be competition between services resulting in an over-concentration on the younger dying person and their family as, for example, the primary health care team and the specialist palliative care team seek to prove that they are most important to the patient. This is another area where self-monitoring and self-awareness is vital, and where teams need to be clear about the impact of particular patients on particular team members.

2.2 ISSUES IN PRACTICE

2.2.1 Access to palliative care

However good the local specialist palliative care service, it is of limited use to a dying person if they are unable to gain access to it when they need specialist input. This is an ethical issue, related to the value of equity. Early hospices were sometimes accused of being predominantly for the middle classes, although there is only anecdotal evidence of this. There is more evidence that palliative care services have not met the needs of those from black and ethnic minorities in the UK. The NCHSPCS, funded by the Department of Health and two large cancer charities, carried out a study to find out if these groups were indeed disadvantaged (NCHSPCS, 1995b). This showed that the Black and Asian communities had a lower incidence of cancer because they had a higher proportion of younger people than the majority population, and therefore might be expected to use fewer palliative care services at the time of the study because these had concentrated largely on cancer, a disease on the whole of late-middle and old age. However, as the minority population ages their need for cancer palliative care will increase. Moreover, the study found that even taking this into account there was an under-representation of these groups in in-patient hospices, where there was insufficient attention to their particular needs. They were receiving care through large hospitals from palliative care support teams or specialist nurses or from domiciliary services.

What can be done to ensure that all groups in the population have an equal opportunity to benefit from particular specialist palliative care services? On the issue of access, each service needs to carry out an audit of referrals if there are any inequitable patterns and what lies behind them. Oliviere (1993) suggests that there may be a need to target particular General Practitioners or referring agents and to develop contacts with local groups. Information about services must be available in local community languages. Once referred, the environment of an in-patient service particularly must be sensitive to cultural factors. This means that requirements for particular food or for privacy must be met without the implication that such wants are unusual or unwelcome. There must be opportunity to practise religious observances. This may mean, for example, providing Muslim patients with the chance to wash in privacy before praying (Neuberger, 1993). Those managing the service and the individual professional both have responsibility to see that there is general information and training available to all staff about different cultural approaches to illness, death and bereavement, on which those in contact with the patient can build an individualized picture of their needs as suggested earlier in this chapter. One way of helping to ensure that a service is respecting the variety of cultures in the local area is to recruit staff from these groups – and not just to the lowest paid and lowest status jobs. Specialist palliative care services in the UK have been slow to make use of the experience of those working in personnel or human resources, and in this field in particular they have much to offer.

Language is often a key area here. The National Council study showed that there were still too many examples of family members, often children, being used to act as interpreters. The result can be both an extra burden being placed on young members of a family and also less likelihood that the professional can be sure that their words and those of the patient are being interpreted accurately. Use of a proper interpreting service, not just of someone from a list of those working in the hospital who happen to speak the language required, is perhaps the most significant indicator of whether a service is really committed to equal access for all cultural groups. This requires proper funding and may require some input of support for those who may be having to interpret painful conversations outside their usual range of interpreting work.

The National Hospice Council study (NCHSPCS, 1995b) has examples of model operational policies in relation to ethnic minority needs and Oliviere (1993) provides a useful checklist. However, it is important to re-iterate that this issue of access and cultural sensitivity is not just about ethnic minorities. There are differences of approach between those living in a working class area of East London and those living in suburban Surrey, not to mention the Welsh valleys. The luxurious furnishings of some voluntary in-patient hospices can make some potential patients feel very anxious about making a mess through incontinence. Locally based services are likely to have a good understanding of the populations they serve, but do need to maintain a constant scrutiny to see that the needs of one section are not being ignored.

Since the publication of the government report, *The Principles and Provision of Palliative Care* (SMAC/SNMAC, 1992), called for the dissemination of palliative care beyond cancer there has been a slow beginning in acknowledging the needs of the elderly dying from other diseases who have been ignored by specialist services in the past. Lloyd-Williams carried out a case note review of all 17 patients who had died within the previous 6 months on the long-stay psychogeriatric wards of a psychiatric hospital (Lloyd-Williams, 1996). She found that many symptoms that needed palliation but did not receive appropriate treatment were recorded and that all patients were in some distress in the last days of their life. Some specialist domiciliary services in the UK are now offering regular support to residential and nursing homes where up to 47% of those aged over 75 may spend the last year of their lives since the reduction of long-stay beds in acute hospitals (Seale and Cartwright, 1994). Staff in these homes are very much in need of training in all aspects of palliative care (Gibbs, 1995). The provision of regular training courses by specialist palliative care staff may be a cost-effective way of improving the level of care in homes without overstretching the domiciliary service. Hospital Support Teams in acute hospitals are also a mechanism for improving palliative care for older people, since they less often limit themselves to cancer patients alone (Smith and Eve, 1994), and those over 65 form the bulk of in-patients in such hospitals. The adaptation of palliative care to the particular circumstances of elderly care is only just beginning.

2.2.2 Handling conflict over cultural issues

Even if the individual professional, and the palliative care service that they work in, is incorporating all the elements of culturally sensitive practice identified earlier in this chapter, conflict may occur over what is acceptable behaviour. Such conflict may occur between staff and patient, staff and carers, within the staff group or between all these different groups. One area where conflict may occur is around issues of autonomy, often involving different perceptions of the role and status of women. Clarke and colleagues (Clarke, Finlay and Campbell, 1991) experienced real distress when faced with a situation where they felt that a Korean patient's wishes were being overridden by her husband, who was insisting on a particular regime of diet and medication, but realized that this might be culturally acceptable for this family. Demonstrating first a willingness to listen to the male carer's point of view and a wish to understand their culture is the first step in establishing that trust without which very little can be done. Recognizing that such attitudes may spring from a wish to value and care for women rather than dominate them, however alien they may seem to the independent female nurse or doctor from a western society, may help. A determination to rescue the patient is only likely to create emotional turmoil for her, even if she is asking for help. The professional can continue to make clear that the service can offer more than is initially being accepted by the male carer, but this can be done as part of a continuing dialogue rather that in a single interview. This is more difficult in emergency situations, but even here the effect on the bereavement of those who survive of any conflict over care must be taken into account. Similarly, Oliviere (1993) tells the cautionary tale of the Indian woman who continues to struggle unaided with housework despite the presence of her husband and adult sons. Staff in the home care team were upset, but to her this was quite acceptable. Careful negotiation with patient and family about how extra help may be offered, using a care management approach which focuses on needs rather than trying to slot someone into an existing service, is appropriate here.

In these situations staff in the team from that particular ethnic group can act as a very helpful bridge. However, it is important to keep the work with the patient and family as the responsibility of the whole team. This needs careful monitoring which should primarily be done by the team leader, but to some extent by all team members. It should not necessarily be the nurse who has grown up in India who is always allocated to the elderly patient from the local Indian community. There may be a danger of overloading that member of the team, pushing them into over-involvement or isolating them. Over-identification of any team member with one side or the other will not produce the best care and requires open, honest but tactful discussion. Issues of teamwork and advocacy will be discussed in Chapter 7.

The conflict may be between the needs of one patient and their carers and those of the rest of the in-patient group. Some cultural groups, for example gypsies, gather together in large groups when someone who is significant in the community is dying. It is challenging to staff to accommodate large numbers of visitors when the usual number is two or three per patient and they may feel they are losing control of the environment. The inevitable increased noise and movement may be upsetting to other seriously ill patients. Some groups may express their grief more openly and loudly. It can be a temptation here for staff from the majority culture, if they are feeling uncomfortable, to restrict the 'unacceptable' behaviour and to do it in a way which implicitly or explicitly condemns it. If the measures identified under the section on promoting access are in place – information and training available to staff, a proper interpreting service – problems are less likely to arise. Preparation and planning beforehand is essential, rather than failing to consider the potential clash until it arises. If the other cultural group is in a large minority locally, keeping a channel of communication open with local priests or community leaders may lead to greater understanding on both sides and enable compromises which are fair to all parties to be worked out. Thinking ahead and admitting the

patient to a single room if death is a possibility will minimize any distur-
bance unwelcome to other patients. However, professionals can also help
those other patients understand what is happening by giving them objective information about the cultural practices of the minority group and,
most importantly, by showing that they themselves treat those practices
with respect.

Sometimes a quick, humorous exchange can stand up for the principle
effectively. A hospice ward sister was accosted by the white relative of a
white patient. 'I'm surprised to see you have people like that in here' he
said, waving in the direction of an Indian patient and their family. 'Well,
we let you in' she replied and went on to make it clear that the service
was for anyone in the community, whatever their colour. If a dying person
is making derogatory remarks about a person of a different culture in an
in-patient setting and does not respond to an initial request by junior staff
to restrain themselves, a senior member of staff should be enlisted to reinforce it. An elderly man constantly referred to a ward housekeeper as
'one of those Irish bastards'. The Charge Nurse went to see him and first
tried to find out why he was so vehement. Hearing that a niece had been
injured some years ago in an IRA bomb explosion provided an explanation, but not a justification for his language in this situation. It was
important to set some boundaries, both for him and to demonstrate to
other patients and staff that everyone would be treated equally. He was
told 'You are entitled to your own feelings, but please keep them private
and treat everyone here with courtesy, as you would wish to be treated'.

2.2.3 Spiritual care

'The whole care and style of what is usually called the modern hospice
movement is productive of spiritual care' (Lunn, 1993). Implicit in the
broad definition of 'spiritual' given earlier in this chapter is that it is to
some degree part of the remit of every member of the team. This is widely
supported by those whose primary area of responsibility it is (Lunn, 1993;
Speck, 1993), yet all too often the place in the notes for recording spiritual issues only has a record of church affiliation. An evaluation of two
specialist palliative care support teams found that they failed to record
spiritual needs (Higginson, Wade and McCarthy, 1992). Spiritual along
with sexual needs seem some of the most difficult areas for professionals
in western societies to enquire about, although nurses regularly ask about
bowel habits and social workers for details of income – both of which are
considered too private in some other cultures. Part of the difficulty is
recognizing when someone is in spiritual distress, part may be due to the
fear that the person who initiates the conversation will be expected to
provide an answer or conversely that there is nothing that can be done
except to listen.

Speck has described some indicators of spiritual distress (Speck, 1993). These indicators may relate to past, present or future. There may be events in this individual's past which are now viewed with guilt or shame, even if they were not at the time. As people approach their death there is often a wish to look back over life and weigh up the good and the bad – to try to understand the painful things that have happened as well as to remember the successes and pleasures. Why did my husband go off with someone else? Would I have been happier as an architect than as a town planner? The highlight of my life was our trip to Israel. This informal reviewing of what has happened in the dying person's life may take place with any member of staff and contributes to that search for meaning in life as a whole and in this present situation. Sometimes a balance sheet may be drawn up. 'On the whole I've had a good life, but I wish I had not quarrelled with my brother and been out of contact for so many years.'

Preoccupation with unresolved issues from the past frequently signals deep-seated distress. The offer of specific counselling sessions or the technique of formal Life Review described in Chapter 4 may be an effective way of tackling this. For those near to death Twycross and Lichter (1993) offer the term 'terminal anguish' to describe a time when because of increasing weakness the patient is no longer able to repress or deny such thoughts and feelings. This is may be shown by increased restlessness, moaning or crying out. If the person is too near death for any real discussion of the anxieties or regrets, Twycross and Lichter (1993) suggests that heavy sedation may be the most merciful response to terminal anguish. However, Kaye warns that this is 'not to be confused with the anguish and distress of many patients who are not yet dying and who need company and counselling, NOT sedation' (Kaye, 1989).

Another indicator is anger, which may be expressed at doctors who are failing to provide a cure, at a god who has not prevented the illness, at those 'who are going to survive when I am not' (Buckman, 1988) 'Behind much of this anger is a desperate need to understand the nature and cause of the illness, together with any part they may have played in bringing it about' (Speck, 1993). Although the person who receives the anger may feel personally attacked, it is important not to respond defensively. Acknowledging with the dying person how frightening it is to deal with the uncertainty of serious illness, saying 'I am sorry that you feel no one has really helped', asking 'Why do you think this has happened to you now?' may begin to open up a calmer discussion which will enable the distressed person to set aside some fantasies or fears. Speck suggests that the subtle change from using the word 'pain' to describe what is felt, to using the word 'suffering' is another sign of spiritual difficulty. This may relate to the perceived meaninglessness of what is being endured, to the loss of control over external events as well as physical functions, to the change in relationships with those previously close that serious illness may bring and the consequent emotional isolation. Jones and colleagues (Jones, Johnstone and Speck, 1989) used cognitive and behavioural methods such as keeping a diary of changing mood to enable greater awareness of positive as well as negative feelings and engender more sense of control by concentrating on one day at a time. These methods may be helpful with those who seem overwhelmed with despair.

It may be issues to do with the future that are causing the distress. Here the identification by Herth (1990) of hope-hindering and hope-enhancing strategies is pertinent. Feeling valued as a person, having meaningful relationships, relief from troublesome symptoms, realistic goals – all contributed to the increase in hope which occurred in the small group of patients she studied as they came nearer to death. All these are areas which professionals can influence and which are, as Lunn says (1993) 'embedded in the tradition of palliative care'. Communicating that this person matters by remembering what they said last time you met, which position they can lie most comfortably in, realism but creativity about what could be achieved this week, can all be part of this. What hindered hope for Herth's patients was the converse of what enhanced hope – feeling unvalued and abandoned, uncontrolled symptoms and no sense of direction. There may also be plans the dying person wishes to make with those who will survive for the future care of vulnerable members of the family – young children or a wife with Alzheimer's disease – or for disposal of their possessions. An important consideration here is to encourage planning that is not too specific. The situation seldom feels quite as expected once someone dies and it may impose a painful extra burden on the survivors if they feel they must either try to live out plans which no longer seem right or ignore a solemn last wish.

Broadening an understanding of the way spiritual distress may show itself is the first step in tackling the problem. The readiness to hear the pain which may be expressed in the variety of ways described above and gently allow the distressed person to talk about what is disturbing is the second. Once it is clear what the issue is there may be a number of choices. It is important not to throw the baby out with the bathwater and, in recognizing that all members of the team have a responsibility here, deny the expertise of the priest or minister of religion who has most training in this area. The issue may be specifically religious. Where it is in the more general spiritual or philosophical arena this member of the team may still have an important direct role if specific allegiance can be humbly laid aside and a readiness to meet the dying person where they are can be achieved. They may also have a useful enabling role. The use of cognitive behavioural methods in the case study cited was carried out by a nurse, but with support from a chaplain and a psychologist. It may be that a member of the team trained in counselling can provide a neutral place to explore troubling issues. Using music or art therapy may be another means – more of this in Chapter 8. The formal Life Review technique to be discussed in Chapter 4 could be used by many professionals. What is important is that there is not unhelpful competition, described by Walter (1994) between nurses and chaplains.

2.3 CONCLUSION

This chapter has outlined some of the cultural and spiritual factors to be considered when working with dying and bereaved people, and offered some ways of approaching problems specific to these areas. Along with the principles and concepts in the first chapter these factors must always be taken into account when working with any individual to appreciate the complexity of the experience for both that person and the professional concerned. In the end this makes situations more comprehensible and understanding is a big step on the path to managing or improving something that feels overwhelming.

Social and health care policy and the development of palliative care | 3

3.1 SETTING THE SCENE

3.1.1 The influences on development

The development of specialist palliative care in the UK was one of the responses of a particular society to a series of social, technological and economic changes in the period after the Second World War. The 1976 Consultative Document *Prevention and Health: Everybody's Business* (DHSS, 1976) charted the conquest or containment by the early 1950s of the common childhood diseases like whooping cough and diphtheria and the huge reduction in the incidence of tuberculosis due to a combination of public health measures and new treatments. Life expectancy for both men and women was rising and death was occurring in old age following a period of chronic disease and deterioration, rather than as a result of infectious disease at any period in the life span. An increasing proportion of the population were over the age of retirement and many more were surviving into their 80s and 90s. The introduction of the National Health Service (NHS) in 1948 made good standards of health care much more widely available, and the development of new drugs and surgical techniques continued to raise expectations about the possibility of heroic cures for the diseases now causing death – circulatory and respiratory disease and cancer (James and Field, 1992). This hope of cure right to the last minute, both by patients and professionals, may have been one reason for the increasing numbers of people dying in hospital, 56% in 1969 (Registrar General, 1969), where high-powered medicine was concentrated.

The domination of high technology medicine was not unchallenged. The Voluntary Euthanasia Society in the UK had been founded in 1935 and a bill was put before Parliament seeking to legalize euthanasia. This was part of a beginning unease, expressed by writers like Illich (1977), about the increasing medicalization of birth and death, which seemed often more concerned with quantity rather than quality of life. Studies in the USA revealed ways in which health care professionals concealed information about their coming death from patients (Glaser and Strauss, 1965; Oken, 1961). Hinton was beginning his influential studies of the dying in the UK (1963), and Bowlby his work on attachment and loss (Bowlby, 1969). The development of psychology and sociology provided different views of the world to the bio-medical, and these began to influence the health and social care systems, drawing strength from their establishment as academic disciplines particularly in the newer universities. A greater understanding of how families operate and ways in which therapy could influence this was emerging from the work of clinicians like Minuchin (1974). The post-war Labour government had encapsulated a national mood which recognized the sacrifices made by all the population in the war and looked for the development of a more equal society. One impact of this was over time less acceptance of hierarchy in society and in health care a growing wish for a more equal relationship between doctors and patients. This was fuelled by the greater availability of information about health and disease through the media of radio and television.

A number of reports in the 1950s and early 1960s had revealed how care in some of the large institutions for the elderly and the mentally ill was little more than 'warehousing' – Townsend's *The Last Refuge* (1962) was particularly influential here. In the cancer care field a survey by the Marie Curie Foundation in 1952 had shown very inadequate support for those with cancer being nursed at home. The establishment of their home nursing support service followed in the 1950s. The increase in life expectancy brought growing numbers of elderly people who needed care, placing a strain on family carers on an unprecedented scale. This was occurring at a time when women of all ages were increasingly seeking employment outside the home, even if only on a part-time basis, making that family care even more thinly spread.

It was against this background that Dame Cicely Saunders worked to raise the money to establish the first modern hospice, St Christopher's Hospice, in 1967 in London. Homes for the dying known as hospices already existed in France, Ireland and in London. It was while working as a nurse at one of these, St Luke's Home for the Dying Poor, that she saw the use of regular doses of oral morphine to control pain, in such contrast to the regimes in most hospitals at the time (Saunders, 1993). It was her achievement to knit together in a unique way so many of the strands previously described. She mobilized the scientific knowledge developing about pain and its treatment and married this with a respect for the individual patient derived from her Christian faith and relationships with patients who had influenced her deeply. The dictum 'Pain is what the patient says it is' represents this wish to stand aside from the power and status of the doctor and to meet the dying person as a partner in care. Implicit in this was the expectation of an open dialogue about the outcome of the disease. Her development of the concept of 'total pain', described in Chapter 1, recognized the inter-connection of all parts of life, including the importance of relationships with carers, so bereavement care is part of the service. Although the focus of hospices and specialist palliative care has been so much on cancer, her vision was of a varied community. St Christopher's has always taken patients with motor neurone disease, and has had a wing for the elderly and a day nursery for the children of staff and local children as part of that community.

She has certainly been a charismatic leader (James and Field, 1992) and Walter (1994) has drawn an interesting contrast between her and another such in the area of death and dying, Elisabeth Kuebler-Ross. Considering the question of how the succession will be managed as each becomes older, he describes the way that Saunders institutionalized this by her support from the start for education and research which has led to a new generation of leaders, most of whom have undergone a more formal training in conventional educational settings. Kuebler-Ross, on the other hand, became more distanced from the mainstream of health and social care than when she was working on her seminal study *On Death and Dying* in the late 1960s in the USA (Kuebler-Ross, 1970). She retains a very personal control over her small Shanti Nilaya organization, has become more mystical in her approach and has 'blessed' only a few to carry on her work.

3.1.2 The process of development

From this beginning came the network of specialist services for people who are dying and bereaved now in place in the UK. Two national cancer charities played a key role in the development. The Marie Curie Foundation's support for cancer care at home has already been mentioned and that was an important ingredient of later developments in home care. In time their homes for cancer patients were remodelled as palliative care units. The National Society for Cancer Relief (NSCR) had, since 1910, made grants to those with cancer to supplement their income. In the 1970s under the leadership of Henry Garnett it saw the opportunity to secure a further improvement in the situation of terminally ill cancer patients by spreading the new model of care developing at St Christopher's. It was a principle of the organization to work in partnership with the statutory services where possible and at this time funding for growth was available in the public sector. NSCR developed an early example of the mixed economy of care by funding the capital costs of setting up 12 Continuing Care Units over the period 1976–82 through local fund-raising appeals and then handing the units over to the NHS to run. For some time NSCR continued to make a small grant to each unit for patient comforts.

With the economic problems of the late 1970s and the ideological hostility of the government in power after 1979 to monolithic statutory services came a change. The statutory sector no longer had the money to fund the revenue costs of large developments. NSCR continued the partnership with the statutory sector but the main focus of its investment became a different type of development, the Macmillan Nurse. The usual pattern was to pay for three years for the cost of employing a specialist nurse which was then taken over by the NHS. The role of the Macmillan Nurse evolved over time from a nurse predominantly offering direct care to that of a Clinical Nurse Specialist with clinical, consultative, teaching, leadership and research functions (Webber, 1993). This evolution moved at a different pace in different geographical areas depending on the level of competence of generalist staff in the area and the precise nature of the contract negotiated with the Health Authority. Initially they were mainly working in the community supporting the primary health care services but posts based in hospices and in acute hospitals, sometimes attached to the growing number of Support Teams, began to be funded. By 1994 over 1200 Macmillan Nurses had been given start-up funding and while the bulk of them were engaged in working with those who were in the terminal phase of cancer, many were offering support to those at an earlier stage of the disease and specializing in particular areas such as breast care or paediatric care. This diversification into working at all stages of cancer, using the word 'palliative' in the broad sense implied by the World Health Organization approach described in Chapter 1, was not uniformly well-received. Some specialists in palliative care felt that it caused confusion about what palliative care was. 'It is important that charities which support cancer care and, in particular, support and facilitate palliative care services should all adhere strictly to the same definition. Sadly this is not happening' (Doyle, 1993b). This was one impetus behind the production of the NCHSPCS Occasional Paper on definitions of specialist palliative care (NCHSPCS, 1995a). Doyle was at that time vice-chair of the NCHSPCS.

Both the Marie Curie Foundation and NSCR, by now known as Cancer Relief Macmillan Fund (CRMF), became involved in education and, to a lesser degree, research in palliative care in the latter part of the 1980s and into the 1990s. Many posts had both a clinical and an educational role. CRMF funded a series of posts in medicine, nursing and social work based in centres of higher education, and developed the concept of the facilitator in general practice, a GP who was supported to devote some sessions to palliative care education. The Marie Curie Foundation put on regular study days, produced a curriculum on ethics, and developed an open learning Diploma in Cancer Care Nursing. The different areas of interest of the two organizations, and the creative competitive tension which this from time to time generated, have been very significant in the development of palliative care in the UK.

However, a parallel and equally important strand has been the part played by local voluntary effort. Another response to the economic downturn and change of government was an acceleration in the growth of new in-patient hospices through the late 1970s and 1980s funded through the efforts of groups of local citizens. Despite the oft-quoted advice of the Working Group on Terminal Care which suggested that there should be a concentration henceforward on developing home care and day care rather than in-patient beds (DHSS, 1980), public support was often more easily mobilized for a building than a service and the number of in-patient units trebled in the 1980s (Clark, 1991). Starting rather later day care did in fact develop too and by 1996 there were over 230 Day services. These did not usually stem from any assessment of need and were often rather unfocused in their aims (Faulkner *et al.*, 1993). Clark's careful study of the genesis of a local service in Newark highlights some of the difficulties for local groups when there are varying views in the community about what type of services should be provided, when resource constraints in the public sector limit support which may have been promised at an earlier stage, and changing professional views of how a service should be delivered cannot be ignored (Clark, 1991). Concerns about the continued revenue funding of some hospices developed by such local groups prompted the founding of the national charity Help the Hospices in 1984 to campaign for greater support from central government and to raise funds to be distributed to voluntary hospices. From 1988 to 1995 a central government grant was distributed to Regional Health Authorities which they in turn were required to allocate to voluntary hospices to promote development.

In practice by the 1990s the mixed economy of care often made it difficult for the lay public, and even professionals, to identify how the service was funded and the different degrees of input from public or charitable sources. The National Association of Health Authorities and Trusts (NAHAT) argued from a small, and not necessarily representative, survey that if the contribution made by the public sector to many voluntary hospices in the shape of provision of free or at-cost goods and services were taken into account, many Health Authorities were supporting their local hospice to a much greater extent than the 50% advocated by central government (NAHAT, 1990). A local in-patient voluntary hospice might over time acquire staff whose salaries were funded by the local fundraising group or by one of the national charities, and then have based at it Macmillan Nurses working in the community whose initial grant had ended and were now NHS funded but managed by the voluntary hospice by agreement. In addition there might be a Lecturer in Palliative Nursing outposted from the local College of Nursing and a social worker funded and managed by the local Social Services Department. The work of these paid staff was supplemented by a group of volunteers, often numerous in voluntary hospices. These were found too in smaller numbers in those services that had started life as NSCR Continuing Care Units, which were also drawing their funds as time went on from ever-widening sources, not just from the NHS.

The rapid and opportunistic development of palliative care services complementary to the existing primary and secondary health care services produced considerable differences of organization and remit between palliative care services. This was at its most varied in relation to Support Teams in acute hospitals, where the model of service ranged from one nurse covering the whole hospital to teams with doctor, nurse, social worker, physiotherapist and chaplain. Some teams made home visits, others handed over to the specialist palliative care community team once the patient was discharged (Eve and Smith, 1994). A number of studies highlighted the lack of clear criteria for referral for palliative home care (Nash, 1993) and this created problems for both the service and the referrer. In her examination of referral patterns to a palliative nursing service Nash found that 68% of those referrals where a reason was given for referral were for 'support'. No indication of what this meant was given. Once referrers were given a checklist of possible reasons to use they were able to be more specific about what they thought the patient and family required. Nash reflects how the advent of contracting with the re-organization of the NHS in 1991 forces a greater clarity about what the service is offering (Nash, 1993).

3.1.3 Future trends

James and Field in an influential article considered the development and future of the hospice movement using Weber's concept of charisma (1992). Their argument is that the early period of separation from mainstream services under the leadership of a charismatic leader – Dame Cicely Saunders – with a few committed followers has ended. With integration has come 'routinization' and in its train bureaucracy. They identify the establishment of the NCHSPCS in 1991, designed to speak to central government with one voice for all the professional and service organizations in the field, as evidence of a more standardized approach. The development of specialist training for different professionals in palliative care feeds into traditional divisions, as may the recruitment of staff who are pursuing a career rather than a 'calling'. They fear that an emphasis on audit and evaluation, where it may be easier to measure the quantitative inputs such as bed usage rather than qualitative inputs such as empathy, could result in an emphasis on physical care to the detriment of essential elements of the hospice philosophy.

Their analysis captures some significant factors in the changing scene in the care of the dying but they do overstate the degree of separation between the early hospice services and the mainstream. As described earlier Cancer Relief Macmillan Fund's developments occurred very much in partnership with the statutory sector. Wilkes, recounting his experience of setting up St Luke's Hospice in Sheffield in the late 1960s, writes 'The Regional Hospital Board agreed that such a unit was needed but said they could not possibly afford to build it. They did agree, however, that if we raised the money to build from private sources they would help generously with the running costs' (Wilkes, 1981). Hillier reports from a survey of terminal care provision in the UK that in January 1980 that there were 22 NHS in-patient units compared with 16 homes run by the Marie Curie and Sue Ryder Foundations and 17 voluntary hospices. There were 10 community and home care teams in the voluntary sector, but 13 community and home care services and five support teams funded by the NHS (Hillier, 1983). Saunders' remark that hospices moved out of the NHS 'so that attitudes and knowledge could move back in' (Saunders, Summers and Teller, 1981) has often been repeated rather uncritically. Initially the bulk of development was in the NHS, it was the 1980s that saw the balance shift to the voluntary sector in the UK.

A complication here is the use of the terms 'hospice' and 'palliative care'. Are they interchangeable? 'Hospice' in the general public's mind is still predominantly associated with an in-patient unit, whereas the term rapidly became used by those in the field to apply to a range of services which might be delivered in the community or in an acute hospital also (Taylor, 1983). With the recognition of palliative medicine as a speciality by the Royal College of Physicians in 1987, the term 'palliative' has been increasingly used to describe services for the dying in an effort to recognize both the different ways the service can be delivered and the integration flowing from the mixed economy of care. Some have also speculated that this is also a way of avoiding the mention of that powerful and final word 'death'. In the shorthand phrase describing the philosophy of palliative care, 'living until you die', the emphasis on quality of life, central though it is, has sometimes obscured the hard fact that this person is going to die.

A particular trend that looks likely to continue is the development of palliative care in diseases other than cancer. In Chapter 2 this has been discussed in relation to older people. Higginson (1993a) has pointed out the scope for greater emphasis on palliative care in the field of HIV and AIDS in the UK. There are some differences – the younger patient group at present still largely drawn in the UK from the gay community or from intravenous drug users, the difficulty of identifying the terminal phase and social attitudes to the disease – but many similarities in symptoms and the need for a holistic approach. While there was specific funding for AIDS services and people with AIDS were on the whole concentrated in urban centres, specialist palliative care services devoted to their needs were developed, e.g. the Mildmay Hospice and the London Lighthouse. Many cancer palliative care services could ignore the relevance of much of what they had to offer to this patient group. A few voluntary hospices feared for the continuance of support from their local communities if they were known to be taking AIDS patients. This picture is rapidly changing as special funding has ended and as many Hospital Support Teams extend the remit of palliative care to patients with any disease.

The introduction of the eligibility criteria for continuing care in the UK in 1996 has implications for palliative care. These were developed by Health Authorities in response to a Department of Health circular (DoH, 1995) in an attempt to distinguish who might be eligible for free health care funded by the NHS and who might be required to contribute towards social care, which is means-tested. Problems arose in the 1990s because of a reduction in long stay beds in hospitals and an increasing reliance on beds in private and voluntary sector residential and nursing homes to provide long-term health and social care, at a time when the requirement for such care was rising because of the increasing number of frail elderly people. This was fuelled by the 'perverse incentive' in the state benefit system which from the mid-1980s provided Income Support to meet the fees for those on low incomes who were cared for in residential and nursing homes, but not for care needed if they wished to stay in their own home. Some people were discharged from hospitals to means-tested care who plainly needed on-going health care, and a report from the Ombudsman criticizing Leeds Health Authority for just such a discharge led directly to the publication of the DoH circular.

While this change was occurring in generalist acute settings, changes were also happening in the shape of the services offered by specialist palliative care in-patient units. As the specialism developed and symptom control continued to improve, in-patient units began to develop rehabilitation programmes which might restore the dying person's functioning sufficiently for discharge to be considered. At the same time the new knowledge about caring for the dying was spreading into the local community as primary health care teams learnt from the advice of specialists. All these factors contributed to a faster turnover in specialist beds and a shorter length of stay. Many hospices began to work to a two week admission for symptom control or respite care and then a planned discharge – part of the routinization and medicalization some commentators identified (James and Field, 1992; Biswas, 1993). However, those who could no longer be cared for in their own homes were often very frail. Plans might be made to admit them to a nursing home with emotional cost to them and their relatives as they contemplated an unexpected move. There might be a financial cost too if they had resources above a certain limit. Many had assumed that the hospice was the place where they would die (Maccabee, 1994). In practice many did in fact die before transfer. A survey of those referred for admission to nursing homes over a six-month period from an in-patient hospice at the end of the 1980s found that only eight out of 18 referred actually moved to a nursing home and only one was alive two months after admission, several dying in the first week after admission (Sheldon, unpublished). Maccabee's small survey (1994) of relatives of those who had died in a nursing home after transfer from a hospice found much dissatisfaction about the care they had received.

The effect of the public disquiet felt about these trends and their impact on vulnerable dying people and their carers is seen in the circular on Continuing Care Responsibilities (DoH, 1995a). In the section on hospital discharge it gives the consultant (or GP in some community hospitals), in consultation with the multidisciplinary team, the job of deciding whether the patient needs ongoing and regular specialist clinical supervision, and thus care paid for by the NHS, because (among a number of other factors) after acute treatment or in-patient palliative care in hospital or hospice his or her prognosis is such that he or she is likely to die in the very near future and discharge from NHS care would be inappropriate.

Already during the period of local consultation on the proposals for the Eligibility criteria the Department of Health warned Health Authorities not to set short, arbitrary time spans on how long someone who was dying might be entitled to care paid for by the NHS. At the time of writing in the first year of operation of the policy the effect on specialist palliative care services is not clear.

Will the future of palliative care be 'masculine' rather than 'feminine' in tone? A focus group study to explore the perceptions and knowledge of lay members of the public about hospice care found that a hospice was 'perceived to be feminine in its general character with an emphasis on softness and tenderness in the form of the quality of nursing care and attention, and amount of time spent with patients' (Hospice Information Bulletin, 1991). The researchers recommended adding what they term a more 'masculine' emphasis on symptom control and research to counteract what they view as the recessive characteristics of softness and tenderness. Walter records his impression that hospices are becoming more masculine with an increase in male doctors and administrators (Walter, 1994). In fact among the doctors who are members of the Association for Palliative Medicine of Great Britain and Ireland women predominate but perhaps it is significant that the first four Professors of Palliative Medicine in the UK were men. Leaving aside the rather sterile debate about which characteristics may be found more often in men or women, there does seem to have been an increase in emphasis on symptom control and research in the 1990s, worrying to some professionals in the field (Kearney, 1992a; Biswas, 1993) who fear that older values will be swamped. Some of this springs from the professionalization described by James and Field (1992). Palliative care has embraced new technology in the shape of syringe drivers, opiod patches and alarm systems, all of which enable dying people to remain longer in their own homes. Old certainties about the inappropriateness of using intravenous hydration for dying patients are being challenged (Dunphy *et al.*, 1995). Saunders' vision was to maintain a holistic and humane approach in partnership with the best of modern therapeutic care, and research is certainly necessary if this fruitful tension is to continue. Further, it is also important to know whether those working in palliative care do actually put into practice the philosophy of care outlined in Chapter 1. Palliative care has been very well supported by the public, often rather uncritically, but this may not continue unless they have evidence that there is real concern to maintain high standards. The limited evaluative studies that have been done show that not all stated goals are in fact achieved. Higginson (1993a) found that support teams were frequently not succeeding in achieving goals on spiritual care or dealing with family anxiety.

3.1.4 The spread of palliative care

Since the foundation of St Christopher's Hospice in 1967 specialist palliative care services have begun to make their appearance in every continent. As Chapter 2 has indicated different cultures and societies will shape the service differently. Much will depend on the economic situation, on the availability and acceptability of pain-relieving drugs, on the levels of existing community health and social services, on the availability of family care, on attitudes to death and bereavement (Ford, 1993). In some countries the locus of development has not been in cancer exclusively. In France geriatricians have taken a lead. In some countries like the USA, professions other than medicine have been at the forefront of development. In India, on the other hand, where the profession of nursing is less respected it has been vital to have medical leadership. The foundation of the European Association for Palliative Care in 1988 demonstrated that much had already been achieved and gave encouragement to those struggling to start. There continues to be a debate about the relative merits of separate specialist services versus integration in existing health and social care systems. In areas where palliative care is at its most developed – in the UK, South Australia, Catalonia in Spain, specialist centres exist as centres of excellence and have a commitment to teaching colleagues in generalist services so that the palliative approach described in Chapter 1 may permeate every area of care.

3.2 ISSUES IN PRACTICE

3.2.1 Over-treatment and under-treatment

With the growing possibilities for treatment and cure in life-threatening disease the potential for disagreement about the right moment to stop treatment becomes ever more complex. The aspect of resource allocation and rationing is becoming more explicitly part of the decision. The case of Child B, whose father refused to accept the decision of Cambridge District Health Authority to discontinue the purchase of treatment for her leukaemia, provides one example of how strongly carers can feel about possible missed opportunities. On the other hand, the legalization of living wills in many parts of the USA, the widespread support for Dr Nigel Cox who killed a patient in pain with an injection of potassium, and the House of Lords acceptance that advance directives can be binding in some circumstances, all reflect a concern that suffering may actually be increased if all possible treatment options are used. What actually constitutes over- or under-treatment is not simply an objective decision, but will depend on individual judgements by all parties about quality of life. There is the problem of balancing the need for more information about new treatments which may benefit other patients in the future with the needs of this patient now. Those with an interest in decisions to stop, fail to start or to continue treatment include the patient, their carers, the different teams involved in their care in in-patient settings and in the community, and society as a whole. The multiplicity of such decisions contribute to forming opinion and standards in a particular society, and professionals cannot divorce themselves from ethical standards in society as a whole (Kennedy, 1981).

Randall and Downie set out the ethical basis for decision making 'it is morally justifiable not to offer life prolonging and life sustaining treatments to autonomous patients... when they are physiologically futile, where their burdens and risks greatly outweigh their benefits, where they may prolong life so that much more unpleasant events which the patient declines to contemplate or discuss are likely to ensue, and where the combination of resource constraints and justice require that treatments should be given to patients more likely to benefit more from them'. They add 'Such complex and onerous judgements are part of professional life in palliative care. The responsibility for them cannot be avoided or passed entirely to the patient' (Randall and Downie, 1996).

But how are such judgements and decisions to be made? Clearly if the patient is able to express a view this must be taken into account. However, human beings can be both ambivalent and inconsistent. A young woman with secondary carcinoma was being treated both by an oncology team and a specialist palliative care team. Her husband was having an affair, she had two children under 5 years old. To the palliative care team she expressed her weariness with her treatment and with life in general. She just wished to spend her last months of life quietly with her children. To the oncology team she expressed the importance of surviving as long as she could for her children's sake and therefore her readiness to continue treatment. Until members of the palliative care team spoke to their colleagues in oncology they were blaming that team for persuading her to continue treatment. These two teams needed to make sure they regularly checked with each other how the situation was developing. In other circumstances it may be that a patient emphasizes different aspects to different members of the same team.

In either situation such decisions need to be widely discussed within the team as well as between teams so that everyone has an opportunity to form a fuller picture, rather than relying on a partial story. It is important for in-patient teams to consult the primary health care team about their views and their knowledge of the patient, particularly if they will be looking after the patient at home during the last period of their life. Senior members in the team, of whatever profession, set the tone in this situation, and they require both maturity and humility to be ready to hear challenges to their own views and engage in discussion. More junior members of the team sometimes fear that if they mount such a challenge they may jeopardize future good references. In practice a well-timed and tactfully expressed wish to understand better the basis of a senior colleague's view is more likely to bring them credit for being thoughtful and discriminating. The views of carers are particularly important, although not more important than those of the dying person, and must be weighed alongside the professional judgements on the merits of stopping, starting or continuing. Unless carers' views are fully and sympathetically listened to, even if they are not the determining factor, and the reasons for the final decision explained, they may continue to make inappropriate demands and may have a more troubled bereavement.

Maddocks (1993) records an interesting approach to 'do not resuscitate' orders which may have relevance for those working in acute settings with dying people. A Select Committee of the Parliament of South Australia recommended that hospitals in South Australia should stop using the negative approach of coded instructions for ' do not resuscitate' orders and should substitute the positive approach of 'good palliative care' orders. They were persuaded by a submission from a hospice which suggested that it should be recorded in the notes that there has been an open discussion with the patient of their clinical situation, and with their permission with family members and staff, and that appropriate management would now be directed towards good palliative care with careful attention to control of discomfort. Suggesting this to the hospital management team and working to secure its acceptance will bring into the open the range of opinion about both palliative care and heroic treatments which bubbles away under the surface in large acute hospitals. The open debate may result in a modification of current policies and a more positive view of decisions not to treat.

Patients or their carers may enquire about the possibility of drawing up advance directives, although Ashby and Wakefield's study (1993) in South Australia revealed that information about this may take a long time to circulate. Only 20% of their respondents believed they had the right to make a living will, although legislation to this effect had been enacted 10 years before the study. Twenty-five per cent of respondents still believed it was illegal to do so. Stern (1993) in her helpful survey of this issue suggests that in the current state of English law this should be done with the advice of a doctor. The House of Lords accepted the position that advance directives should be binding upon doctors if there is clear evidence that they were intended to apply in the precise circumstances that the patient is in. Since those exact circumstances may not occur, Stern recommends an advance directive should be drawn up, or reframed, at a time when both the patient and the doctor are aware of the prognosis and the treatment options available.

3.2.2 Requests for euthanasia

The purpose of this section is not to debate the merits of the case for or against euthanasia but to look at some of the issues professionals need to consider when they are faced with a request for euthanasia. It is important to be clear that there is a distinction between assisting a mentally competent patient to die and good medical practice which ceases futile life-prolonging treatment, although the line may be a fine one. Perhaps surprisingly the wish for the option of euthanasia has been shown to diminish as people become more sick. An Australian study (Owen *et al.*, 1992) of the views of 100 cancer patients at all stages of the disease showed that whereas 50% of those at an early stage wished to have the options of suicide or euthanasia, there was a significant decline in the proportion of those with late-stage carcinoma who felt the same. Hunt and colleagues (Hunt *et al.*, 1991) were interested in the incidence of requests for euthanasia in dying people. They collected staff's statements at death audit meetings in a palliative care unit about patients' spontaneous expression of requests for a 'quicker terminal course' over two years. Only 6% of patients made serious requests, though a further 18% made more indirect allusions to the possibility. The researchers acknowledge that patients may have been inhibited from asking, recognizing that the setting might be hostile to the idea, and that staff might for the same reason have recorded only the most obvious requests.

Given that only relatively few may seek this option, how is it to be handled? The law of the country clearly sets a boundary where euthanasia is illegal, but it is not helpful to stop the conversation by mentioning this as a first response. A serious request will usually indicate deep despair and suffering, and hopelessness. Much more rarely it will be a testing of the attitudes of the person asked, for fear that euthanasia may be practised without consent. In either case the question must be asked – 'What has made you feel like that?' – and the reason given explored further – 'Tell me more about that'. Cole in his discussion of four case histories of people who asked seriously for euthanasia reflects 'Sitting down to discuss the reasons behind the request enables the care-provider to find the appropriate responses to hidden agendas rather than become embroiled in legal and ethical considerations at the outset' (Cole, 1993). As the discussion continues the professional may be able to give reassurance that no measures will be taken to prolong life, and that there are good possibilities for controlling pain and other distressing symptoms.

Fear of loss of control and of pain are two major factors behind such requests. The value placed on autonomy has been influential in the changes in practice in the Netherlands which now permit voluntary euthanasia in some situations, and seems to be an important factor in the greater frequency of such requests from people with AIDS. However, Seale and Addington-Hall (1994) provide a reminder that an important aspect of loss of control is the dependence that frequently accompanies it. They drew on material from the Regional study of 3696 people dying in 1990 and from the 1987 study by Seale and Cartwright (1994), both of which used relatives' reports about the experience of the last year of life. The relatives were asked both whether the dying person had ever asked to die sooner, or for euthanasia, and what their own view was about the timing of the death. From their data the researchers drew the conclusion that different causes of death create different patterns of distress and dependency. Those with cancer were often distressed and it was the fear of pain which was an important factor in cancer patients in the study requesting euthanasia. They were less dependent and when they were dependent it was often for relatively short periods. For those with other conditions such as Alzheimer's disease or respiratory disease, and for their relatives, dependency was more important than pain. Specialist palliative care has concentrated on good symptom control as the main remedy for preventing people wishing for euthanasia and this clearly stems from its base in cancer care. In extending its remit beyond cancer there has to be more attention paid to issues of dependency. The next section on making home care possible has an important bearing on this, since many people feel less dependent in their own homes rather than in an institution, although a key factor in this may be the extent to which they have to call on their family for help and how acceptable this is to them. This may be particularly an issue in elderly care.

The reassurances that it is possible to give about pain control and respect for their wish to be in control may enable many who request euthanasia to withdraw, as Cole (1993) shows. However, there will still be some who are not shaken. Since the Suicide Act of 1961 it has not been illegal to commit suicide in the UK, only to assist someone to do so. It may therefore be important to say gently that it is not possible to agree to help carry out the act, but not to imply that efforts will be made to stop that individual from committing suicide, unless the dying person is judged to be suffering from clinical depression. Palliative care services need to ensure that they have good advice from mental health specialists on this issue (Kissane, Finlay and George, 1996). Any refusal to agree to carry out euthanasia, at the end of a discussion on the principles outlined above, must be communicated in a way that does not make the dying person feel rejected. Assurances should be given that despite any disagreement about this issue, the team will continue to offer their skill and experience and will strive to respect the patient's wish to remain in control in all other areas, provided these do not infringe the autonomy of others.

3.2.3 Making home care possible

For many years it was an article of faith in palliative care that home was the best place to die – best because that was the opinion expressed by dying people in a number of studies (Dunlop, Davies and Hockley, 1989; Townsend et al., 1990). It chimed in too with the drive towards delivering services in the community rather than in large institutions evident in all areas of health and social care in the 1980s and 1990s. However, Hinton (1994a) has shown that the issue is more complex. In his prospective study of a random sample of adults with carers referred to the St Christopher's Hospice Home Care Team between August 1984 and July 1986 he found that at the point of referral all patients preferred to be cared for at home but as they neared death an increasing preference emerged both in the patients and in their carers for in-patient care. By the last week of life most were admitted, if only for the final day or two, and only 27% died at home. Following reorganization of home care services, attachment of a social worker to the teams and improvement of day care services over the next few years the proportion dying at home rose to 34%. Hinton's research and that of others suggests that it is far more frequently relief of relatives that prompts admission, than uncontrolled symptoms (Doyle, 1980), although it is not always clear what role uncontrolled symptoms may have played in the carer's distress. It may be easier for the professional referrer to attribute the need for admission to the carer's burden rather than their own difficulty in managing care. In-patient palliative care units recognize in some of their referrals the phenomenon of primary health care team distress.

However, it does seem that carer burden or lack of a carer are very important factors in bringing about admission to in-patient care in hospice or hospital, or to residential or nursing homes. What do carers require to enable them to continue caring? Thorpe (1993) has listed a number of elements:

- Adequate nursing support.
- A night sitting service.
- Good symptom control.
- Confident and committed general practitioners.
- Access to specialist palliative care.
- Effective co-ordination of care.
- Financial support.
- Terminal care education.

What is adequate nursing support to one family is not to another. When the wealthy owner of flourishing mobile home business was dying of cancer his wife was well able to afford the provision of 24 hour nursing care at home. Neither this nor the regular visits of the palliative care team were able to help her contain her dread and fear at what was happening, and the prospect of him dying at home was unbearable. He was admitted to the hospice some weeks before his death. A family of three daughters in the same village wished to care for their dying mother without assistance, apart from a regular telephone call from the palliative care team. Negotiation of the right balance of services for *this* patient's and carers's needs is what is at issue. For some carers the provision of domestic help to enable them to continue the personal care of the dying person is the most important, for others the availability of a sitter so that children can be fetched from school by a parent rather than a school friend's mother.

The introduction of care management gives the potential for developing services more tailored to need, but it is still vital for professionals to carry out the negotiation in a way that does not imply that family members should behave in a particular way or be expected to undertake certain tasks. For a daughter in one family toileting her mother may be quite routine, for another daughter in a second family seeing her mother even partly naked may be impossible. It is important too to be sensitive to the invasion of intimacy and privacy which even wanted and carefully delivered services can bring. A widow at a bereavement group related how she cried bitterly the first time her dying husband was washed and put to bed by a paid carer. She had asked for the service, she needed it, but it was concrete evidence of how her husband was deteriorating and how much she was losing. She resented that she could no longer do it. In the UK an increasing number of Hospice at Home services are developing including both professional nurses and untrained paid carers, supplementing the care that Social Services Department home carers and Marie

Curie nurses already provide, to give the intensive 24 hour support which may make it possible for someone to die at home without completely exhausting their carers.

Confidence is one of the keys to home care – confidence of both the dying person and the carer. A 55-year-old married woman had well controlled symptoms following a hospice admission and was relatively mobile although easily fatigued. Her husband was out at work all day. She resolutely refused to consider discharge from the hospice and infected him with her terror at being alone most of the day with just the episodic visits from the home care service that her condition was seen to justify. She was gently encouraged in the hospice to make a number of visits home, always at the weekend when her husband was there, with the assurance that she could return whenever she wished. From one such visit she returned with the decision that she was now ready to be discharged, overriding the concerns of her husband who was now more anxious than her. She remained at home for some months, mostly on her own, until just before her death. Making haste slowly, and giving a real assurance that a bed would be there if needed, enabled her over time to reassemble her own coping mechanisms. Insisting on discharge as soon as symptoms were controlled would in the long run have been more costly in terms of the emotional stress on patient, carer and hospice team, and in financial terms. A holistic approach must mean weighing feelings and fears as important as physical symptoms.

Twycross and Lichter (1993) point out the crucial importance of doctor availability in generating the confidence that can maintain home care. Most studies of home care (Addington-Hall and McCarthy, 1995; Hinton, 1996; Seale and Cartwright, 1994) show that a substantial proportion of relatives wanted GPs to visit more often than they did, particularly as death approached. Such visits were seen as evidence of concern and valuing the dying person, rather than being necessarily required for symptom control. It may be useful for other professionals in the team to help their medical colleagues understand how much their presence can be valued, not just their knowledge. Such visits need not take a great deal of time. They may also contribute towards fewer demands on the primary care service from the surviving carer whose bereavement may be less problematic because they have felt well supported over the time of the death.

Financial and resources issues are still very much underestimated by many professionals as a source of difficulty when someone is dying at home. Higginson, Webb and Lessof (1994) have shown that in London dying people are more likely to be admitted to in-patient care from areas classified as socially deprived and further national study has found wide variation in the proportion of those dying at home, often but not invariably, linked to deprivation (Irene Higginson, personal communication). Addington-Hall and colleagues (1991) found that 27% of their sample of dying people in an inner London borough did not have a carer. Other studies show that people are much more likely to die at home in rural rather than urban areas. So the range and quality of services from area to area will be responsible for some of the variation in numbers who die at home. However, finance has both practical and symbolic aspects. When the Attendance Allowance became available to anyone in the UK who was judged likely to die within a certain period it provided a very welcome additional sum for those struggling with paying increased heating and tele-phone costs at a time when the income of both dying person and carer are likely to be much reduced. However, it also had a symbolic impor-tance in providing some official recognition that the serious illness of this individual mattered. Again this is part of holistic care and every team needs someone with a full understanding of the system of state benefits and any voluntary grants that may be available to the dying person and the carer as much as its needs someone with counselling skills or physio-therapy training. This is most often provided by a social worker attached to the team who can contribute other knowledge and counselling skills as well, but could come through contact with a local welfare rights service, or through the Citizens' Advice Bureau. Some palliative care services employ a social work assistant to look after this aspect of care. Beck-Friis and Strang (1993) report that 42% of carers of the patients served by their hospital-based home care service in Sweden exercised a right to receive an allowance corresponding to their net salary. They saw this as an important factor, along with prompt provision of necessary aids and equipment, the promise of a bed when necessary and 24 hour on call support, in making it possible for 89% of the patients of the service to die at home in contrast with the 85% usually dying in hospital in Sweden.

3.3 CONCLUSION

With the development of specialist palliative care services against a back-ground of economic, social and organizational change has come a far more flexible and needs led service for those who are dying and their carers. Maintaining the high quality of this and ensuring the diffusion of pallia-tive care concepts and practices through the whole health and social care system is a continuing task. Part of the quality lies in an appreciation of the individual's response to their own death and their view of what makes up quality of life for them. The next chapter will consider these issues.

The individual facing death | 4

4.1 SETTING THE SCENE

Can we really understand the feelings of the dying, their anguish, their contentment, their joy, their despair? Are there some common elements experienced by all or most dying people? To enter fully into the feelings and experience of another human being is impossible even when both parties are in very similar situations. For a professional, a well person, perhaps at a very different time of life, to attempt to understand something of the individual mixture of feelings of a particular dying person is very challenging. Yet to offer holistic care this does have to be attempted. Acceptance of the concept of total pain demands it. The contribution of cultural and spiritual factors to the dying person's experience was outlined in Chapter 2 and this chapter should be read with these in mind. In particular the importance of the meaning attributed to the experience, discussed in Chapter 1, is of key importance, determining so much of the dying person's attitudes and behaviour. After some of the different models of psychological responses to dying have been described and analyzed, the theoretical aspects of denial will be looked at in more detail and quality of life for people who are dying will be considered.

4.1.1 Psychological responses to approaching death

A number of writers have sought to identify the psychological responses of those who are facing the end of their life. In the second half of the 20th century the ideas of Elisabeth Kuebler-Ross have been immensely influential. A psychiatrist working in a Chicago hospital in the 1960s, she interviewed over 200 dying people and from this developed her distillation of their experiences, 'the stages of dying' (Kuebler-Ross, 1970). She herself did not claim that she had produced a 'complete study of the psychology of dying' or suggest that all dying people would have the same responses or follow a particular order of response. What she did say was that she had found some common elements to the experience of those she interviewed. These were:

- Denial.
- Anger.
- Bargaining.
- Depression.
- Acceptance.

Her ideas emerged at a time when there was beginning to be a recognition that the dying had been ignored. She herself contributed a great deal to this new interest and the establishing of a dialogue with the dying. However, the 'stages' were seized on by those professionals desperate for a guide through the pain of those they wished to help and rapidly developed into a prescription that all dying people should progress through them to the goal of acceptance. They met the need identified by Benner (1984) for new professionals to seek the support of guidelines and rules in dealing with the complexity of human problems. In time practice experience and the expertise derived from it allows a more creative and flexible approach. Kastenbaum (1975) has pointed out that Kuebler-Ross's study was descriptive, and that 'virtually every operation that might have been performed on clinical information for conversion into research data has been neglected'. There is little information in the book about the age, gender, ethnic origin, position in the lifespan of the individuals she talked to, or the effect of the disease and environment of the hospital on them – all of which may have had an impact on their responses. Walter (1994) hypothesises that she may have seen predominantly younger people (though younger people are usually less well represented in hospital populations than older people) and that her formula is likely to be more applicable to younger people dying of cancer. Without more information about her study it is hard to be sure. Certainly Weisman and Kastenbaum (1968) carried out a retrospective study, 'a psychological autopsy', of the experience of a group of chronically ill older people before their deaths and found patterns of adaptation to impending death ranging from continued activity to withdrawal. However, the limitation of their study is that it was based on the observations of staff after the death rather than on contact with the older people themselves. As indicated in Chapter 2, there is some evidence to show that older people approach the idea that they may die differently from younger people, although it is not clear how much of this applies in the UK, and more detailed work needs to be done to understand the experience of older people who are actually terminally ill.

Others who have attempted to describe the experience are Buckman, Shneidman and Corr. Shneidman worked mainly with younger people and produced the idea of 'a hive of affect, in which there is constant coming and going of feelings' and a vacillation between acceptance and denial (Shneidman, 1973). Buckman drew from his clinical experience and proposed a potentially three-stage model:

- Facing the threat.
- Being ill.
- Acceptance.

In the initial stage the individual may show a mixture of reactions, characteristic to that individual and which may include fear, anxiety, shock, disbelief, guilt, humour, hope or despair as well as those identified by Kuebler-Ross. There are similarities to Shneidman's 'hive of affect' here. He describes the second, chronic stage as one of flat emotions and frequently depression, with resolution of the elements of stagë one which can be resolved. The third stage of acceptance he does not regard as essential provided the patient is not distressed, is communicating normally and is making decisions normally (Buckman, 1993b).

Corr takes a slightly different approach (Corr, 1991–92), developed in response to the limitations of a rigid interpretation of the 'stages'. If the style of the 1970s was to look for stages, both in dying (Kuebler-Ross) and in bereavement (Murray Parkes), the style of the 1980s was to identify tasks for the dying (Corr) and for the bereaved (Worden). His theoretical model is rooted in the ideas developed by Lazarus and his colleagues on stress and coping. His view is that any model should fulfil four criteria: it should enable understanding of all the variations in the situation studied; it should empower by emphasizing options; it should encourage sharing and participation; it should guide care providers. He suggests that there are four tasks for dying people:

- To satisfy bodily needs and minimize physical distress in ways that are consistent with other values.
- To maximize psychological security, autonomy and richness in living.
- To sustain and enhance those interpersonal attachments significant to the person concerned and to address the social implications of dying.
- To identify, develop or reaffirm sources of spiritual energy and in so doing foster hope.

The influence of the concept of total pain is evident. Corr's objective is to provide a descriptive model but, even though his is very broadly drawn, there is still an element of prescription, which is perhaps unavoidable, in the very notion of 'tasks' and in the choice of the values which underpin the model.

In these different approaches there is a good deal of common ground. Denial, fear, acceptance and anger are mentioned by most of them. Most writers identify a complex mixture of emotions that arise in no particular order. As others have built on or reacted against the interpretation of the Kuebler-Ross stages it has become clear how much there is still to understand. Age is probably one of the crucial factors in determining reactions, but what about gender? Research by Brunning and Hesselink (cited in Munnichs, 1987) in the Netherlands on the affect and behaviour of 191 older people dying in a nursing home found that of those able to respond, more women than men were calm and accepting, more men than women were anxious and afraid. Is death universally feared? Some argue that it is – this would certainly be a Freudian position – and fear of death has been held to be the force behind religion (Walter, 1994). Others have pointed out that, for example, Judaism has not always been concerned with the afterlife (Bowker, 1991). All those who have produced models of psychological responses have come from Western Europe or the USA, so the models may not fit those from other cultures.

Models are useful in that they may alert those who wish to help to emotions that they had not expected that people who are dying would experience. They offer some sort of framework, though preferably a loose one, at a time of pain and suffering. Models are unhelpful if they produce rigid expectations and prevent the individual's real experience being heard or make the dying person feel inadequate because they are not conforming to some 'right' way to die. Kastenbaum (1975) suggests that the reason for the popularity and wide dissemination of the 'stages of dying' is that it is so difficult for professionals to be in daily contact with the suffering of dying people and their families that they seek a 'delimited, coherent, orderly sequence' to contain their anxieties and sense of chaos. If this is a possibility then it is important to look for other ways of managing which do not circumscribe the dying person. Chapters 7 and 8 will have material which may help in finding such ways. Walter (1994) comments that the 'stages' model has been more widely taken up in the USA where the interest in death, particularly in the shape of death education, came earlier than in the UK. A critical view of it has certainly been more prevalent in recent years among specialists in palliative care, but its accessibility makes it still very well-known and it continues to shape the thinking not only of many of those working in general social and health care settings, but of some carers and, on occasion, of the dying person.

4.1.2 Denial

There are many misconceptions about denial. This section will outline both what it is and what it is not. Ways of working with people in denial will be considered in the Issues in practice section. There are two different theoretical approaches to the concept of denial. Freud, who first described it, viewed it as an unconscious mental process – a defence against the anxiety produced by an external threat. Those of the Freudian school have often viewed denial as pathological because it blocks or distorts reality. The second theoretical approach is that of Lazarus, for whom denial was a coping mechanism – a way of avoiding the stress of physical illness – and so not necessarily pathological. So whichever theoretical basis you prefer might affect how denial is dealt with in practice. Denial is not suppression, which is a conscious process – 'I don't want to think about it'. Disagreement with the professional's view is not necessarily denial. A woman who had a very firm conviction that prayer would bring about a cure was not denying. She had a different view of how the world worked from the doctor who was treating her for the secondaries from her breast cancer. Sadly in the end his forecast proved more accurate, but it did not dent her conviction and that of her relatives that it was possible for prayer to be effective in such situations, even if it had not been in hers.

There are cultural elements in denial. There is a widespread popular view in western Europe and the USA that a 'positive attitude' to cancer will help to prevent recurrence, drawn from research on different survival rates for patients with different psychological approaches to the disease. Although subsequent research (Mulder *et al.*, 1992) has made it clear that the links are less firm than once thought, such a popular belief might lead to suppression at the very least and might well contribute to denial. The Jewish view of the importance of maintaining hope could be an influence for people of that faith.

Relationships with professionals can also be a factor. Ross and colleagues (1992) studied the different approaches of doctors and nurses working in a cancer centre in the USA. They found that doctors were much more ready than nurses actively to allow denial, and that patients behaved differently with different caregivers. They concluded that denial is an interpersonal as well as an intrapersonal process. A man who had received a trailblazing new treatment from an eminent surgeon was told he would have many years of life, yet seemed to have continued symptoms. The Palliative Care Team treating the symptoms felt his life would be much shorter, but he held firmly on to what he had been told. Eventually as the disease progressed he acknowledged to this team that he now saw that he would soon die. However, he confessed that when he went for his follow-up appointments with the eminent surgeon that he maintained the fiction that he believed he would survive, as he felt he had let the doctor down by failing to respond to the treatment.

4.1.3 Quality of life

Ensuring that the dying person experiences the best possible quality of life is the over-arching goal of palliative care. But how is this to be defined and is it possible to measure it? Both these are necessary if professionals are to know whether their goals for care are valid, both on an individual and service level. Moreover, in developing any new treatment in this field assessing its impact on quality of life is essential. In Ahmedzai's useful short review (1993) he suggests that quality of life has three theoretical components: the absence or presence of subjective feelings of pleasure or happiness, normative ideals of activity or performance and the preferences of the individual. Calman has put forward the view that what is important is the gap between the person's actual condition and the state he or she would ideally wish for (Calman, 1984). The greater the gap between the person's present state and wished-for state, the less satisfactory is their quality of life. This approach deals with the situation where someone with what is assessed by others as a very unsatisfactory quality of life says that it is perfectly acceptable to them at the time. Popularly known as 'the Calman gap', it provides an important perspective for work in palliative care and may prevent fit professionals thinking that they can know what is important to someone with life-threatening disease.

Many scales for measuring quality of life have been devised and increasingly new tools are being developed specifically for those with people who are terminally ill (Ahmedzai, 1993). One aspect of this development links to 'the Calman gap' and recognizes that only the individual dying person can say what quality of life means to him or her (though any assessment has to take into account the frequent reluctance of patients to criticize those who are currently treating them). Rathbone and colleagues demonstrated this neatly when in-patients admitted in a seven-month period to a voluntary hospice were asked to identify and grade problems as they perceived them and to grade problems previously identified by the medical and nursing staff (Rathbone, Horsley and Goacher, 1994). The doctors and nurses were good at picking up pain and immobility as problems, but much less good in relation to psychosocial problems. Fifty eight per cent of patients identified problems not seen by the professional and 52% of these were psychosocial. This reinforces the importance of starting with the dying person's views. There remains the difficulty of how to determine whether quality of life is good enough for those who are too unwell or unwilling to complete questionnaires or visual analogue scales – 27% of those at Rathbone's hospice. Chapter 5 will consider the issue of whether carers can be used as proxies in this situation.

4.1.4 Communicating with people who are dying

Since open and honest communication is one of the principles of palliative care, considerable attention has been paid to communication and to communication skills by specialist practitioners, teachers and researchers in the field. The influence of this principle and the practice based on it is one of the contributing factors to the increase in openness with all cancer patients recorded by Seale and Cartwright in the 18 years between their two studies of the year before death (Seale and Cartwright, 1994). They found that for cancer patients the proportion who knew what was wrong with them had risen from 29% in 1969 to 73% in 1987 and those who knew they would certainly die had risen from 16 to 44%. In those suffering from other diseases there was little difference in the proportions over the period. Moreover, unless the professional knows what is really concerning this particular dying person or carer it will not be possible to offer the holistic care which addresses total pain. There are ethical, contextual and technical issues to be considered in the area of communication.

One ethical issue concerns the right to information. Does the information about the disease and its progress belong to the doctor, the person who is dying or their closest carer? The principle of autonomy requires that the dying person is given information which allows them to remain in control of their situation. The Patient's Charter in the UK gives the patient the right to a full explanation of the range of treatments available and this implies that that person also has at least some information about the disease. Certainly contemporary professional practice is on the whole very different from that recorded by Hinton in his work in the 1960s (Hinton, 1967) when doctors seemed to have the control. However, there are still ethical challenges in practice. What if the relative insists that she will not let the visiting nurse into the house unless she promises to conceal the truth? What if it seems that the patient does not want to be fully informed? These issues will be discussed in the Issues in practice section.

The context of the communication is now being given much more attention in the palliative care field. In the concentration on developing communication skills in the 1980s (Maguire, 1985; Maguire and Buckman, 1985; Maguire and Faulkner, 1988) the importance of the environment and the role of the dying person were neglected in favour of an emphasis on the contribution of the professional. Now Wilkinson (1991) has shown, for example, the influence of the ward sister on the ability of nurses in an in-patient setting to use communication styles which open up discussion. Jarrett and Payne (1995) have pointed out that the other party in the dialogue, in this case the dying person, is making choices about what to communicate of which the professional may be unaware. They may decide that this nurse is not the right one for them to confide in or that this morning the ward is so busy they will confine themselves to superficial exchanges. The importance and subtle influence of cultural factors for both professional and the person being communicated with is gradually being better understood. The increased amount of time that dying people spend at home may also help the development of a more equal balance. It is more difficult to ignore these factors if the conversation is taking place in the dying person's home. Professional training for doctors and nurses is now having to adapt to a more community focused service.

The importance of paying attention to particular communication techniques to enable the dying person to present their anxieties and fears has been well documented (Maguire, 1985). Building on the models of counselling such as that of Egan (1994) attentive listening, the use of open questions and empathetic summaries are now forming part of the training of the majority of professions in social and health care. How to approach giving the dying person or a carer 'bad news' will be considered in the Issues in practice section. But communication is not just about counselling techniques. The non-verbal elements of communication continue to be the most powerful and the major part of any encounter (Birdwhistell, 1970). Attempting to secure sufficient privacy to make the person feel safe by drawing the curtain round the bed in hospital, or negotiating whether a student should be present at a home visit, sitting down to model the partnership of the relationship, using touch but only lightly at first until it is clear what is comfortable for this person – all these will communicate much about the tone that the professional wants to set for the conversation. Research has shown the influence of a homely environment in making in-patients in a hospice feel secure and valued (Neale, 1989). The use of cognitive and behavioural therapies is developing with people who are dying (Moorey and Greer, 1989) although more evaluation of their effectiveness is still required. The potential of these techniques for working with depression and fear will be considered in the Issues in practice section.

4.2 ISSUES IN PRACTICE

4.2.1 Ethical challenges in communication

As we have seen in Chapter 1 a principle of palliative care is that people have a right to information about their situation so that they can exercise autonomy. However, there are people facing life-threatening illness who are clear that they do not wish to know the details of what is happening to them. 'I leave it all to you, Doctor...' 'Just discuss anything about what is going to happen with my daughter, she knows what is best.' Randall and Downie (1996) suggest that there can be no absolute right to remain in ignorance. Those who are HIV positive, for example, have a duty to safeguard any sexual partners and can only do so if they have appropriate information. However, unless there are issues about protecting the welfare of others (some of these will be discussed in the section on working with denial), the principle of autonomy permits the dying person to choose to remain in ignorance or with a limited explanation. Sometimes it is evident that the dying person has a very good idea that something undesirable is in store and that they prefer to keep their distance from emotional pain. The professional's wish to be open should not override this, but there is a responsibility to check from time to time that the dying person has not changed their mind. The issue of the carer who wishes to protect the dying person by keeping bad news from them will be considered in Chapter 5.

4.2.2 Breaking bad news and eliciting concerns

Finding out what way an individual who presents with a potentially life-threatening illness would prefer any information or decision-making to be handled is the responsibility of that member of the team whom they first consult. In most circumstances in the UK this will be the GP. This is the point at which it can be discussed whether the person wants the results of any investigations to be given to them alone, to be conveyed when both they and their main carer are present, or discussed only with someone else. Failure to carry out this piece of work, and to communicate it to anyone who will subsequently be treating or working with the patient, can cause uncertainty for those who come after and may result in the sick person being deeply distressed by not being treated in the way they wish. Once it has been done it can set the tone for how any bad news about diagnosis or prognosis may be shared.

Maguire and Faulkner (1988) have identified some useful techniques for delivering bad news, and provided that these are adapted to the cultural context and used taking into account the issues discussed in Setting the scene, they remain a helpful guide. Their view is that to give bad news too abruptly may disorganize the person psychologically and cause the defence of denial to be brought into play. They recommend a stepwise approach which starts with a warning shot, e.g. 'We now have the X-rays and unfortunately they do show a problem. Would you like to know what we think?' This gives an opportunity for the person to signal whether they are ready for more detail or not. If they then request more information, a short explanation avoiding any technical terms should be given and an empathetic statement added: 'I'm afraid we have confirmed that you have multiple sclerosis. This is a disease which affects the nerves and I would be glad to give you more detailed information if you wish. I'm afraid this may be very disappointing.' The person then has a chance to express something of the many different emotions they may be feeling, fear, panic or even relief that it is not something they dreaded more. There can then be some exploration of any knowledge about or experience of the particular disease. When some of the feelings and concerns have been talked about, the professional may turn to what can be done if the person seems to wish to continue. 'Even though we cannot cure the disease, there are many things we can do to reduce any problems from it.' The professional has to make the judgement how much the sick person can take in at any one time. It is good practice to ask at intervals whether they have heard enough for today and whether they would like to arrange another session when they have had more time to think things over.

The heavy responsibility for giving bad news falls most often to a doctor in hospital, but there are many examples of current good practice which involve other team members. A nurse or social worker may sit in on the interview so that they know what was said, and can be available for the patient or the carer who wants to ask questions about what was said. They may follow up with a home visit within the week (Ackerman, personal communication). Frequently patient and carer are so stunned just after the interview that they cannot immediately think of the questions that flood in once they are home. Another approach to helping with later questions is to offer the patient a tape of the consultation to play at home. This has been shown to be much welcomed by patients (Hogbin and Fallowfield, 1989).

Where the situation is one of giving news of deterioration in an existing illness the dying person may be half expecting it because they are experiencing some symptoms, although they may be using defence mechanisms like denial or suppression to deal with their anxiety. The dying person may initiate the conversation 'I'm getting worse, I'm not going to get better am I?' Here it is important to understand what their real concerns are and not to make assumptions. To avoid them feeling a sense of frustration at not receiving a straight answer it is important to reassure them that you will respond to the question, but first you would like to know what makes them ask it. This will ensure that you and the dying person start from the same point.

4.2.3 Working with denial

When there is concern expressed either in the team or by a carer that the dying person is in denial, there are a number of steps to be taken. First there should be a clarification that it really is denial and not one of the other mechanisms outlined in the Setting the scene section. Second, a discriminating assessment of what is being denied is required. Weisman (1972) has helpfully distinguished between three different types of denial in terminal illness:

- Denial of the primary facts of the illness.
- Denial of the clinical significance or implications of the illness.
- Denial that the illness will end in death.

Each might require a different approach. The third step is to ask – whose problem is it? Is it the professionals' problem because they are working from a rigid theoretical view which specifies that everyone should die openly accepting their own death? This is an issue that needs to be tackled through an open discussion of everyone's views, perhaps at a training session or team away day, where it can be detached from the heat of the moment. Teaching about denial should be part of every professional group's qualifying training, whatever their area of special interest, since the issue does not only appear in the care of the dying. However, for those specializing in palliative care a discussion about it could be a useful part of an induction programme, so that any variety of views in the team is clear. The principle of autonomy must lead to a respect for the right of dying people to use the mechanism of denial, provided that the denial is not harming themselves or others. Another form of professional problem with denial may be for a team member who has become very committed to this particular dying person, and now finds it very difficult to contemplate that all measures have failed and that the person is close to death. This needs to be tackled with gentleness and understanding by colleagues, recognizing that for all of us there are particular patients about whom we find it more difficult to remain objective

Is it the carer's problem? Are they really anxious to have the opportunity to talk openly with the dying person to ask forgiveness for problems in the past, to tell them how much they have valued and will miss them or to ask their advice on plans for the future? If the dying person is firmly turning away all attempts by the carer to open up discussion then the appropriate strategy is for one of the professionals in the team to give an opportunity to the carer to talk in confidence about what is concerning them, perhaps encouraging them to put it in the form of a letter to the dying person which will not be delivered. Anna, a daughter who was quite close to both her parents, wanted very much to talk openly with her dying mother about what was happening. Both parents resolutely refused to talk about the possible bad outcome with her, despite her attempts to do so, though the team suspected that husband and wife were both aware of what was likely. She was offered a series of sessions with the team social worker in which she talked about her feelings and about her relationship with her mother, and this seemed to help her contain her frustration at not being able to talk to her directly.

Is it truly the patient's problem? It might be so in two ways. Denial of the facts of the illness or of the implications of the illness may lead to a refusal to accept treatment on the assumption that, for example, there has been a mix-up about the diagnosis. This is more likely to happen at earlier stages in the illness than at the stage when specialist palliative care becomes involved, unless the team is one that does see patients at all stages of the disease. Ness and Ende (1994) suggest some approaches that may be helpful. They recommend working with the grain of the patient's defence using positive reframing, saying, for example 'Your determination to get better is a real asset in helping us to improve your situation'. Simple clarifying statements and questions may help to demystify what is seen as an overwhelming threat. 'Even when illness causes severe pain at any stage we now have many different ways of tackling pain, and can do so much more effectively than in the past.' Empathetic listening and responding to specific concerns, using the techniques described by Maguire and Faulkner (1988) already mentioned may make the person feel safe enough to let the painful reality come into their conscious thinking. Ness and Ende's final suggestion is using confrontation, but not in an aggressive way, and giving the person an opportunity to reflect on the contradiction. 'You are telling me that you will be fine once you have had a holiday, but what I see is some one who is less well than the last time they saw me.'

The second way denial may be the patient's problem is if their behaviour is showing considerable distress but they are continuing to deny that they are concerned or that there is anything serious wrong. They may be very restless and unsettled, they may be extremely irritable, they may have persistent nightmares. Once the possibility of any adverse drug reaction has been excluded, denial may be considered as a cause. Here an elliptical approach may have a chance of success. Kearney (1992b) gives an example of the use of guided visualization which allowed a young man to work on the fears which were increasing his pain, but without explicitly discussing them. Art or music therapy may provide other ways of communicating what may be too dangerous to allow into consciousness. These approaches will be discussed further in Chapter 8.

Is the problem one of vulnerable dependents for whom plans need to be made if the person is going to die? Is the dying person a single parent caring for young children, or for someone with learning disabilities or the partner of a frail and confused older person? This may be one of the very few occasions when an attempt has to be made to open up discussion with the person who is denying about the seriousness of the situation. Mavis had five children all under the age of 12. Her husband was in prison for harming the children. Even when he was released he was unlikely to be seen as a suitable person to look after them. Mavis had secondaries from breast cancer, and was already having considerable support in looking after the children from her sister and from the Social Services Department. She recognized that she was seriously ill but denied that she would die from her disease. As she became more disabled it became clear that permanent plans needed to be made for the children so that they could begin the process of making the transition to living with others which would be completed when she died. She had to be involved in these discussions and give permission for any steps that might be proposed. Buckman (1988) suggests using the 'What if?' approach to try and help the person in denial to maintain some distance from the painful truth. So saying 'We are working to try and improve the situation, but what if the worst happened and you were no longer around to look after your children, who would you want to be involved? May we have permission to work on that basis?' may provide a way of moving forward.

4.2.4 Working with anger

Just as when working with denial the professional needs to be clear what the patient is angry about. Buckman (1992) attempts a classification of different sources of anger, dividing them into abstract, unfocused anger such as anger against loss of control or against fate, and anger which focuses on something specific like the doctor, family members who will survive or God. However, sometimes it seems reasonably obvious that the abstract, existential anger has been displaced onto a more concrete object. In dealing with anger there are some important principles to consider. Anger may be destructive but it can also be energizing. Many of the voluntary groups in the palliative care field have been started because of someone's anger, because of their determination that no one should have to experience what they have done. So the professional's first aim should be to reduce the destructive force and, if at all possible, enable the anger to be directed more positively. Two dangers are that of becoming patronizing, on the one hand, and defensive, on the other. Anger may well be a common response to the realization that life is short, but if this is too glibly acknowledged by a professional, the reaction is likely to be an intensification of the anger, not a feeling of being understood and accepted. The uniqueness of this individual's situation and of their anger is what is important.

It is hard not to be defensive when you or a colleague are being criticized. A difficult situation is that where you may genuinely feel that wrong decisions have been made. To have the honesty to say 'Things have not gone as everyone would have hoped. I wish it had been different' is less likely to produce a litigious response than a shuffling or attacking retort. It is possible to find the words to express regret without formally accepting blame. It may be important to speak to the feelings underlying the anger – recognizing how unfair life can seem, understanding that anger may spring from fear.

Equally it is essential to demonstrate that however angry someone is, whether that anger is a reasonable response to incompetence or a 'rage against the dying of the light' (Thomas, 1952), there are boundaries to be observed. Physical violence is never acceptable. Words that are everyday for some groups in society are experienced as insulting by others, so it is important to temper any reaction by understanding this. Nevertheless no professional should be expected to tolerate a sustained verbal attack, though a brief explosion may be overlooked. Explaining in a calm but firm manner that you would like to understand more about how the dying person or carer sees the situation and inviting them to sit down with you to discuss it in a quiet place may help to defuse the situation. If angry behaviour or words persist in an institutional situation it may be important to state calmly and clearly that you will summon help if it continues.

In someone's home it is a sensible precaution to ensure that you are nearest to the door and to make it clear that you will leave unless the person becomes more rational. Prevention is better than cure, and if you expect that you are going to meet an angry person then taking a colleague with you may be another way of helping to maintain the boundaries.

4.2.5 Working with depression and sadness

One challenge in working with people who are dying is to decide when their unhappiness at what is happening to them is a reasonable response to their situation and when it has become the clinical disorder of depression. Buckman (1992) lists nine symptoms of depression (Table 4.1) and suggests that at least five must be present for two weeks, one of which should be depressed mood or loss of interest or pleasure.

A difficulty with including physical factors such as fatigue or weight loss when screening those who are dying is that these may be due to the underlying disease rather than to a clinical depression (Faull *et al.*, 1994). Breitbart and Passik (1993) identify a pervasive hopelessness accompanied by despair and suicidal ideas as being most indicative of depression in this group.

Pharmocological treatments have an important place in the treatment of a frank depression, but cognitive therapy is now being explored as an additional therapy for those who are depressed and as a means of helping those experiencing overwhelming sadness and despair. This therapy is directed at helping with the control of intrusive thoughts and unpleasant feelings by using such techniques as cognitive reframing, visualization and relaxation. It is well established with cancer patients at earlier stages of the disease (Moorey and Greer, 1989) but Cocker, Bell and Kidman (1994) showed in a pilot study that women with advanced breast cancer had less depression and anger following an programme of cognitive therapy. In Chapter 2 the potential of the therapy with those experiencing spiritual distress has been

Table 4.1

1. Depressed mood or irritability
2. Markedly diminished interest or pleasure in almost all activities
3. Significant weight loss or gain, or decrease or increase in appetite
4. Insomnia or hypersomnia
5. Psychomotor agitation or retardation
6. Fatigue or loss of energy
7. Feelings of worthlessness or excessive or inappropriate guilt
8. Diminished ability to think or concentrate, or indecisiveness
9. Recurrent thoughts of death or recurrent suicidal ideation

Reproduced with permission from Buckman, R. (1992) *How to Break Bad News: A Guide for Health-care Professionals*, Macmillan Medical, London.

described. The boundaries between depression, sadness and spiritual distress will always be difficult to determine objectively since the interpretation will depend on cultural factors and the theoretical approach of the professional concerned. So alongside any pharmocological treatment there should always be a supportive approach which continues to empathize with the emotional pain and assures the dying person that they will not be deserted even if there is no curative treatment. A 40-year-old man with a long history of alcoholism and now with cancer of the lung was an in-patient in a hospice for symptom control. He had no home, and his possessions could be put in a cardboard box. He was hopeless and over-whelmed with sadness. The doctor put him on anti-depressants, the nurses cared for him and he was seen by the social worker about his need for a home on discharge. A place in a local hostel or a bed-sitting room were the possible alternatives and filled him with despair. The social worker attempted to stay alongside his despair but also to maintain her own faith in the coping skills that he had demonstrated in difficult situations throughout a turbulent life. After about two weeks he met her one morning with the comment 'Right – when are you going to sort out that place in the hostel for me? I'm ready to make a move now'. It was impossible to know which intervention in the whole package was most help, but all of them showed him that his emotional pain was taken seriously by the members of the team in their different ways.

One important principle is to avoid premature or unrealistic reassurance. This can be quite a temptation when confronted with depression and despair. Maguire in his review of psychosocial interventions to reduce affective disorders in cancer care (1995) makes it clear that premature reassurance is likely to prevent the disclosure of all the concerns that the sick person is feeling. Only after the professional has acknowledged the person's distress at the situation and made sure that all their concerns and feelings have been heard, will reassurance be heard and accepted. Too often they will have been inappropriately reassured in the past by family and friends who are trying to deal with their own feelings of impotence and misery as much as with the dying person's feelings.

4.2.6 Life review

Faced with approaching death it is common for the dying person to look back over their life and review what they have achieved, what they regret, what they still wish to accomplish. Opening up such a discussion with some one who is dying will contribute to holistic care by giving the professional a more complete understanding of this person's unique life course. However, a more formal approach to life review may be a useful intervention for those who seem to be in spiritual distress, who are torturing themselves with guilt or are particularly angry or irritable. It may have an impact on the experience of pain. Walker and her colleagues (1990) studied elderly people living in the community and experiencing pain, not all with cancer. They found that those with regrets about the past were both more likely to be depressed and to experience poor pain control.

Life review was initially developed in the field of elderly care following Butler's influential paper (1963) which drew from Erikson's work on life stages (1965). In particular it related to the final stage of ego integrity versus despair. Erikson suggests that each individual progresses through eight life stages and at each stage there is a potential for a positive resolution which contributes to the development of maturity. Those who achieve ego integrity have an assured sense of meaning and order in life, while those who do not may fear death. Butler's view was that reminiscence and the life review which may develop from it could provide a way of integrating past and present, and he saw that it had potential not just for older people, but also for those facing their own death.

Increasingly more formal attempts are being made to harness the power of this process in palliative care. Lichter (1993) in a hospice in New Zealand has trained volunteers to help patients complete oral or written biographies, and Pickrel (1989) has used life review techniques with this group in the USA. Lester in the UK has built on Haight's well-researched intervention of structured life review with older people in the USA (Haight et al., 1995) and has adapted it taking into account the possible needs of those who are dying (Lester, 1995). A structured questionnaire covering childhood, adult life and the present can be worked through over three sessions with a professional. The dying person has the list of questions before the sessions and chooses which areas to focus on. In the pilot study the participants showed a marked improvement in their life satisfaction and a reduction in emotional stress. The formal structure seems to contribute a particular sense of seriousness which adds weight to the process. It also emphasizes that the dying person is in charge, since they choose the areas for review.

Life review is an individual task, but a more deliberate use of reminiscence in day centres can provide another route to helping individuals to integrate past and present, and may often provide important insights to the professional team about the life experience of those in the group. Members of the group are invited to focus on a particular period – perhaps the Second World War – or on a topic like work, and are invited to bring to a reminiscence session some object relating to the subject and to talk about its significance. Considerations of safety and confidentiality are important in both reminiscence and life review. Individuals and the group as a whole must feel that what they contribute will be treated with care and need to consent if what happens in the life review or reminiscence group is to be shared with others.

4.2.7 Groups for patients

Informal reminiscence often takes place at support groups for dying people. Such support groups are well-established in cancer care in general and a randomized controlled trial by Spiegel *et al.* (1989) even suggested that participation in such a group might prolong survival. They are now beginning to develop in palliative care settings. Professionals have sometimes feared that such groups will challenge their authority and have therefore felt ambivalent about encouraging them. Of course much informal sharing of experience and emotions goes on between dying people as they meet in out-patient clinics, day hospitals and as in-patients. However, such situations may not always feel safe enough to express the worst fears about the manner of death or the most critical comments about the care being given and the informal group is very subject to interruption. A formal group which has regular sessions and protected time for meetings encourages the development of trust and concern among group members. The role of the professional is both practical and enabling. First it is to help the group to meet by providing a comfortable room, ensuring that those who wish to come can physically come and negotiating with other staff that the group will not be interrupted during the time allotted. Second, it is to make sure that the group starts and finishes at the times agreed to avoid any embarrassment for those group members who are dependent on others to come and go. If it is an open group then new members will need to be recruited and welcomed. The manner of the welcome will contribute to a third task – to help to create a climate of respect for the views of all members of the group by remaining neutral in any discussion, and making room for someone to express a point of view different from that of the rest of the group by saying, for example 'Many of you seem to see it this way but there may be others here who have a different experience'. All these parts of the professional role will contribute to developing the sense of safety without which group members will not dare to express their questioning and fears.

It is perhaps not surprising that support groups for dying patients occur most frequently in day care settings. The dying person is living in their own home, is clearly still relatively more autonomous than someone who is an in-patient but is regularly gathering together with others with similar problems, and any troublesome symptoms may be reasonably under control. In this setting the group members are not dependent for every activity on professionals so it may be easier to question and explore their situation. Each group can be encouraged to find the right balance for its members between sharing experiences, seeking information and discussing emotions and relationships. The patients' group in the day centre at St Christopher's Hospice has developed in a particularly autonomous way (Carter, 1994) with members initiating the most painful topics and giving advice to each other on problems in a very much more direct fashion than staff could.

One issue that inevitably arises for such groups is the frequency with which group members become more ill and die. Professionals can help the group to be open about this by updating the group on what has happened to those who are not attending but they may also play a role in helping the group to devise strategies to cope with this. This might involve a short moment of silence at the start of the group for someone who has died since the last meeting, or planning that the group has some fun as well as some serious moments. Group members will certainly have their own creative ideas about how to handle this issue and should be encouraged to discuss them.

4.3 CONCLUSION

This chapter has picked out some of the more common issues that face professionals working in palliative care with those who are dying. But no book can cover every situation. The dying person is a partner in the process of care who has their own strengths, as well as areas where they need help. The professional brings their particular knowledge and skill to the encounter, but they bring themselves too. It is in that delicate nego-tiation and balancing of what each partner contributes that the challenge and stimulation, pain and pleasure of working with people at the end of their lives is found.

Carers and families – the time before death | 5

5.1 SETTING THE SCENE

This chapter will look at the issues that may confront carers and families before the death. Chapter 6 will look at bereavement in more detail. However, in practice there is not such a neat split, since what goes on before the death has a considerable impact on the experience of bereavement. This chapter should be read too against the background of chapters 2 and 3. Cultural expectations of the roles, rights and responsibilities of family members, and the way these are enshrined in social and health care policies help to shape the experience for carers. However, each individual family also builds their own patterns of relating and expectations derived from, or in reaction to, the experience of past generations. A key challenge for professionals is to lay aside their own expectations of how family members should behave to each other, and attempt to understand the family that is before them. This does not mean setting all boundaries aside. Each state has laws which set limits to the ways adults may behave to children or to each other and these provide a framework for palliative care, just as for other areas of health and social care.

5.1.1 The changing nature of the family

Hall and Kirschling (1990) define families as 'interrelated, interdependent, interacting complex organisms, constantly influencing and being influenced by their environment'. This definition seems at first sight slightly arid, but it does encompass the wide variety of family structures developing at the end of the 20th century, and includes both heterosexual and homosexual partnerships. Such 'complex organisms' may include close friendships and the potential for clashes between the different elements in the situation is considerable. High rates of divorce, but high rates too of second marriage or stable partnerships have produced both split families and reconstituted families, particularly in the UK. Over the last 10 years an increasing proportion of families are headed by a single parent, most often a woman. These are phenomena that professionals are working with every day but as yet there has been very little research examining the particular difficulties which may face carers who are part of such complex family situations and are also caring for someone who is dying. In the 19th century a similar number of marriages ended because of the premature death of one partner and there were frequently second marriages, but these situations did not so often have the rage and hurt that may be part of divorce. Colin Murray Parkes has described this as the 'monsterization' of the divorced partner in contrast to the idealization which may occur of the partner who has died. Forty-year-old Adam was dying. Some years before he had had an acrimonious divorce and since then had seen little of his son, now aged 12. He was anxious to see the boy before he died to try to explain that he still loved him, but his former wife felt very bitter and refused to allow the boy to visit his father. This was very painful not just for the man himself but also for those professionals caring for him. However, it is also not uncommon for some divorced partners to set their differences on one side and for the healthy partner to take on the care of the other, even having them back to live in their house to care for them.

Despite their increasing levels of paid employment women continue to provide the majority of care for those who are dying although there is some evidence that for those who are dying of cancer the care may be more widely shared around the family. This may be because the period of dependence is usually shorter and because of particular perceptions of the disease (Neale, 1991). Hunt's study of specialist palliative care nurses supporting carers at home showed that the nurses in the study accepted that it was to be expected that gender and the closeness of the kin relationship were the determinants of who became most involved with caring. It also demonstrated that, despite the announced aim of palliative care being to consider the patient within their family as the unit of care and to give meeting carers' needs a high priority, this was interpreted in a particular way. When carers attempted to put their own needs centre stage the nurses in the study gave support directed at enabling the carer to continue caring, rather than give up (Hunt, 1992).

5.1.2 Conflicting demands for carers

Carers may well find themselves juggling the demands of care-giving, employment and other dependent members of the family, such as young children. In her qualitative study of 14 carers looking after 10 dying people being visited by a hospice home care programme in the USA, Hull

(1990) found that a group of major stresses for the carers were around relating to other family members, friends and personal care aides. They might receive conflicting advice from different family members about how to care for the dying person, and have to manage this tactfully. There are both positive and negative aspects to receiving social support (Kirschling, Tilden and Butterfield, 1990). If a carer judges that the emotional price to be paid for receiving support from family members is too high, it may be refused even though it is offered and needed. Elizabeth, caring for her elderly mother who lived with her, really needed a break. She said 'Maureen my older sister is a widow and is free to come and stay – but she has always criticized me and made me feel inadequate. I'd rather hang on until the respite care that has been arranged in a couple of months time'. In Hull's study (Hull, 1990), personal care aides who were unreliable created rather than relieved stress, as carers had to reorganize at short notice their own work or study routines. There is an ambivalence about the support of professional helpers. Their help is valued, but it is hard to be constantly on show, especially if it is not made clear when they are likely to come, and they arrive just after the carer has settled the person who needs care and has put her feet up for a desperately needed rest.

Another conflict identified by the participants was the need to put their own lives on hold. This was exacerbated by the regulations of the American hospice programme in the study which required that the patient was never left alone, but this is an issue for carers even where there is no such demand. For younger carers this may mean foregoing job opportunities, particularly difficult in a world of employment where short-term contracts are increasing and employers may penalize those who take time out or appear less committed by not renewing their contracts. The widespread stretching of the sickness benefit scheme in the UK, where GPs may agree to sign off a carer as sick when in fact they need to take time out to care, is one sign of this, and of the lack of adequate financial recompense for carers. For older carers this may mean ignoring warning signs of their own health problems. While Mary cared for her husband at home as he was dying of stomach cancer she found a lump in her breast. She chose to ignore it until after he had died. By then the cancer had spread and she herself needed hospice care, much to the distress of her two daughters. Studies of carers have shown the bad effect of caring on the health of this predominantly elderly group (Levin, Moriarty and Gorbacy, 1994). One local Carers' Group produced a report which asked statutory agencies to recognize that 'a certain amount of sleep is a human right!' (Eastleigh Carers' Group, 1992). Hinton's prospective study of a cohort of patients of St Christopher's Hospice from referral until death found that by the last interview before the death 17% of their carers were seriously depressed and 14% were very anxious, suffering more emotional distress than the dying person (Hinton, 1994b).

5.1.3 Support for carers

Neale (1991) identifies six areas of activity which define what support might be for carers:

- Practical help with household tasks or personal care for the dying person, equipment or home modifications.
- Enabling help which provides advice and information on what services are available and assistance in securing them.
- Respite care which may be offered by an admission to a home, hospital or hospice, or by providing a sitting or nursing service in the home to relieve the carer.
- Financial support to maintain an income for the carer as well as meet the extra everyday costs for heating, telephones and food when someone is ill at home.
- Palliative care for the dying person which offers indirect help to the carer by, for example, securing good symptom control or regular monitoring of changes in the situation.
- Psychological and emotional help directed specifically at the carer, which for a minority come through carers' groups or formal counselling, but much more often from friends, neighbours and family members.

All these may contribute to tackling the social and psychological pain of both the carer and the dying person, and most of them have been discussed in Chapter 3 in relation to making home care possible. As Neale points out it is co-ordination that is often the difficulty and other studies (Addington-Hall, 1991; Sykes, Pearson and Chell, 1992) have shown the problems caused by the late arrival of equipment and the failure of professionals to advise on the availability of financial support. Fifty eight per cent of those in Sykes study were not claiming state benefits to which they would have been entitled. However, an attempt to improve co-ordination by employing two nurses to act as 'service brokers' or case managers in a randomized controlled trial in the London borough of Wandsworth showed only a very few significant differences in outcome for the carers and dying people in the intervention group compared with the control group, although bereaved carers who had received the service were significantly less angry when they thought of the death (Addington-Hall et al., 1992; Raftery et al., 1996). The trial did reduce the use of resources to achieve the same result, mainly because of reduced length of hospital stays in the intervention group. The researchers suggest that skilled professionals, such as the nurses in this case, may be less effective case managers than non-professionals because they will tend to be diverted into using the other skills that they have in preference to concentrating on co-ordination.

Twigg (1989) has distinguished three types of relationships that social care agencies may have with carers: as a resource for the patient or client, as a co-worker or as a co-client. If they are seen as a resource then as long as they keep going any of their own needs will not be considered. If they are seen as a co-worker, then their co-operation is valued and the aim of the social care agency is to maintain them as carers. If they are seen as co-clients then their needs must be given equal weight with the patient or client and this will involve considering what services will specifically meet their needs. The approach of the Department of Health in the early 1990s (DoH, 1989), enshrined in legislation and departmental guidelines, was to view the carer as a co-worker and for this reason to take some notice of the particular needs that they voiced, but not to suggest to them that there might be the possibility of help with anything that they did not mention. This was the approach taken by the home care nurses described by Hunt (1992), although one of the principles underpinning palliative care, as we have seen in Chapter 1, is that the carers needs should be treated as of equal importance – that is that they should be treated as co-clients. This perspective may be particularly difficult to maintain in a climate of reductions in the funding available to local authorities such as occurred in the mid-1990s.

5.1.4 Sexuality

At first sight it may seem unusual to consider this issue in the chapter on families and carers, rather than in the chapter which focuses on the individual. It is important not to assume that someone who does not have a partner does not have a sexual identity or wishes or regrets about their sexual life (Fallowfield, 1992). However, for most people their sexuality is expressed in relation to others, even if sometimes only in fantasy. Sexual relationships and behaviour may be deeply affected by life-threatening illness – for better or for worse. Gilley's sensitive paper shows the range of responses that may occur, from the couple who could incorporate the wife's physical care for her husband into their intimate relationship to the couple who had not touched each other for so long that a request by the dying husband that his wife should brush his hair was perceived by her as an intolerable intrusion (Gilley, 1988). It may be very difficult for staff meeting couples in institutional settings to guess at which end of the range any particular couple lies. Community staff visiting at home may have more clues to help them decide.

It is well established from many studies in the cancer field (Anderson and Van Der Does, 1994; Fallowfield, 1992) that the disease and its treatment affects the sexual experience of patients and their partners, and that the issue is very seldom tackled by professionals, even where the cancer is one that affects the sexual organs. Their concerns may be around altered body image or altered sexual function, or both. Wright's careful study of how a cancer hospital dealt with this issue with a group of patients with gynaecological cancer found a recognition by staff that sexual issues should be discussed, but a lack of confidence in how to go about this which resulted in patients not having appropriate information and suffering anxiety (Wright, 1996). They made judgements about who might have sexual concerns based on assumptions. A married woman of 70 was excluded by staff from the part of the research into patient experiences on the ground that she was too old and a sex worker was not offered the chance to participate. Despite the inclusion of an item on sexual issues in the patient record it was seldom completed. If this failure to tackle the issue is generally the experience for heterosexual couples, it is all the more true for homosexual couples – except in services for those with AIDS and HIV where open discussion is more the norm. Some ways of opening up discussion about sexual issues will be considered in the Issues in practice section of this chapter.

5.1.5 How similarly do dying people and their carers perceive the situation?

There has been considerable research and debate around the question of whether carers' views on the effectiveness of treatment, the adequacy of services, the degree of distress caused by physical symptoms and the dying person's understanding of their situation can be a reliable guide to what the dying person themselves may feel and think. Many early studies, most notably the two national studies of aspects of the last year of a structured sample of people who had died, used carers or relatives as informants (Cartwright et al., 1973; Cartwright and Seale, 1994). In those studies it was because they were carried out after the death, but others have been concerned to spare sick people the burden of responding to questionnaires or taking part in long interviews. Cartwright and Seale themselves tried to explore how reliable their informants might be (Cartwright and Seale, 1990), and subsequently other studies have looked at this more closely. Field and his colleagues reviewed previous research (Field et al., 1995) and concluded that, if the self-ratings of patients and their carers are compared, carers are likely to overestimate pain, dependency and disability. Dying people report themselves as more positive about their situation than the carers. This may relate to the gap between expectations and reality – the Calman gap – discussed in Chapter 4. Spiller and Alexander (1993) discuss some of the possible explanations for the discrepancies over emotional state found in their study. Carers might be projecting their own distress onto the patient, or assuming that the patient is feeling as they think they would in the same position. Patients might be in denial (but we have seen the difficulties of diagnosing this in

Chapter 4). They might be more truthful with the researchers than with their carers for a variety of reasons.

Field *et al.* (1995) point out that one explanation for the differences in some studies is likely to be that patients and carers were making their assessments at different times, patients at varying periods before the death, carers sometimes at quite a time afterwards. Their own study attempted to overcome this by asking patients and their carers about the same events and experiences one month before admission to a hospice and during the admission. They also found that carers reported more depression and anxiety and more distress at physical symptoms than the patients did. There was more agreement about what help was needed and about the acceptability of the care received. They conclude that, with some caveats around the small size of their sample and the need to be rigorous in deciding exactly what is being assessed, it is possible to use the carers' view as a substitute when interviewing a patient would be too distressing for them. However, perhaps the most important observation that they make is that 'At a global level, the question of whose account is true may be a fruitless one, since both patient and carer accounts are prone to bias. Indeed both accounts may be a true reflection of differing accounts of the experience of dying. The dying patient may have different relationships with particular individuals and thus impart differing viewpoints to each. Also when people are dying (and even when they are not) their views may well be changeable and inconsistent' (Field *et al.*, 1995). The search for objectivity is spurious in this context. This reinforces the importance of treating the views and needs of carers as seriously as those of the patient, and of understanding the ways those in close relationships affect each other (Jenkins, 1989). The implication is that if carers feel that those they care about are in pain and distress this has to be tackled with them, offering them opportunities to discuss the situation. Spiller and Alexander (1993) point out too the danger of challenging a patient's defences inappropriately on the basis of information from a carer.

5.1.6 The needs of children facing bereavement

Walter (1994) has described how in the neo-modern approach to death there has been a sea-change in the way that children facing bereavement are dealt with. No longer are the old ways of silence and concealment seen as appropriate. Children should be included in open discussion about what is happening. This change has to some extent been built on research. Rutter (1966) was one of the first to show the damaging effect that the life-threatening illness of a parent has on many aspects of the child's life and children who have been informed about their parent's impending death have been found to be less anxious (Rosenheim and Reicher, 1985, cited in Black and Wood, 1989). However, it results as much from general changes about openness in society and a less hierarchical approach to children in general, and a particular view of children's rights to information. Not that this approach is universal. Robin was 3 years old when his mother died of breast cancer. She had been determined that she was going to live – she could not entertain the idea of leaving her son – but she died rather earlier than expected during a hospital admission for symptom control. When the social worker went to see Robin's young father a few weeks after the death she enquired how Robin had taken the news of his mother's death. He responded that he had not told him yet and did not think it necessary. Probably he would say something before he went to school. Like many parents he was acting from a mixture of motives – a well-meaning intention to protect the child from emotional pain, a wish to hide from his own misery and a belief that Robin was too young to understand about death.

In fact children as young as 3 years old do have the potential to begin to put together an understanding of what the word 'death' means. To do so children need to grasp that when someone is dead they are gone and will never come back, that their body has changed and can no longer feel or move, and that everyone will die in time, even they themselves. A number of studies (Kane, 1979; Lansdown and Benjamin, 1985) have shown that by the age of 3 children understand that death exists and that it means separation, by the age of 5 many children will have taken on board all the different components of the concept, and by the age of 8 or 9 virtually all children will have done so. What makes the difference between the 6-year-old who has a full understanding and one who does not is both the opportunity the child has had to experience a death, perhaps of a pet or of a grandparent, and the way that experience has been handled by adults. Helping parents and children to talk about a coming death in the family and avoiding some pitfalls will be considered in the Issues in practice section.

Children become adults, but they do not cease to be children of their parents, and an interesting study of psychological morbidity in the families of patients with cancer provides a reminder of the emotional pain for adult children of older dying parents (Kissane et al., 1994). As the researchers observe, this is a group that is often overlooked. In their study over an 18-month period of all adult cancer patients of an oncology service with a given prognosis of less than one year and with adolescent or adult children they found clinical depression in 28% of the children. They were significantly more angry than either the patients or the patient's partner – 25.7% of them being angry as against 8.9% of patients and 13.1% of spouses. The researchers comment that this might be due to anticipatory grief, but might be because they may have less easy access to information about the disease and about the progress of the patient than the patient's partner.

5.2 ISSUES IN PRACTICE

5.2.1 Mapping the support networks

Using genograms or drawing up a map of their social network demonstrates how the dying person is part of a particular system of relationships – both influencing and being influenced by them. A genogram is an expanded family tree that records not just the facts of births, marriages and deaths but adds detail which is important for the current situation. This might be about past illness in the family or about where family members live or their employment. Such details can alert the caring team to points of stress or where support may be located. Most patients will enter fairly readily into drawing up their genogram if the professional explains the need to understand the whole situation. It is easy to update. For some this information is too painful to share and it cannot be demanded. It may only emerge over time in the context of a trusting relationship with a particular professional. Societal and political factors may affect willingness to give the information, e.g. in immigrant families where there are real or imagined anxieties about the possibility of deportation for family members. An example of a genogram is given in Figure 5.1.

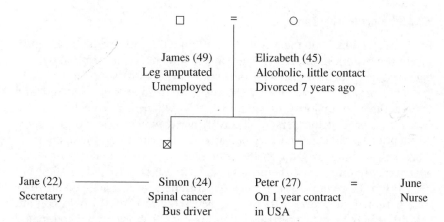

Figure 5.1 A genogram.

Another approach is to develop a plan of the network surrounding the dying person which shows where links within and beyond the family exist, and the nature of the relationships. An example for the same situation as in Figure 5.1 is given in Figure 5.2.

The richness of the information generated through these methods can help to make a reality of a holistic approach to care for the dying person,

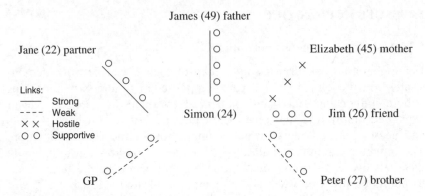

Figure 5.2 A family network.

and an appreciation of the stresses and strains for family members which should lead to improved support for them. Setting out the genogram may also help the family to see that it has faced problems in the past and found ways of solving them or reassure them that though one individual dies the family goes on.

5.2.2 The protective carer

Every professional will meet from time to time the carer who refuses entry to the house unless there is an agreement to conceal the truth about the diagnosis or prognosis, or who buttonholes the ward sister and tries to extract a promise of secrecy by the team. It is important to understand that in the vast majority of situations this will spring from love and a concern to protect the person who is dying. It would, however, be unrealistic not to recognize that very occasionally the carer may be acting from more self-seeking motives to do with securing some financial or other advantage. In either case the professional's first task is to understand what lies behind the request. It may relate to a remark of the sick person years before that if they ever had this particular disease they would commit suicide. It may be the experience of another relative or friend who seemed to deteriorate as soon as the truth was known or remained fighting until the end because they did not know the truth. It may be the carer feels that it would be too distressing for themselves if the situation were openly acknowledged. It may be more difficult to detect the rare situation where the motive is to secure some advantage. Evidence about this may emerge over time from other carers or from observation.

Once there is a better understanding of reasons for the anxiety the professional can express their own empathy and concern for the troubled carer: 'I can see that his previous episodes of depressive illness are bound to make you worried'; 'The fact that her mother died in such agony must be on your mind a great deal now she has the same disease.' It may be possible to give reassurance about improved control of pain or other symptoms, or about the sort of services now available to support the dying person or the carer. Such reassurance should be specific and tempered with reality; 'We can almost always reduce pain nowadays'; 'In this area we have a night sitting service which can come in up to four nights a week.' Only when the professional has demonstrated that the carer's concerns have been heard can the next step be taken. The professional can gently put before the carer the problems that are likely to arise for them if the dying person asks for the truth and they are unable to give it. Since the course of the illness will probably demonstrate that the professional has lied, or at least been economical with the truth, the trust of the dying person might end up being severely shaken. Carers may fear that the professional will be so intent on honest and open communication that they will be determined to dump the truth on the dying person without any sensitivity. Hopefully the earlier demonstration that this professional is empathetic, in the way they have taken the trouble to listen to the carer's anxieties, will have already begun to allay these fears. Reassurance can be given that the professional will not initiate a discussion about diagnosis or prognosis, but will only respond to questions from the dying person and will even then use the approach described in the Issues in practice section in Chapter 4 to discover what the person is really asking before plunging into an explanation which is not required.

5.2.3 Meeting sexual needs

Since this seems to be a particularly difficult area for professionals to discuss, but one that dying people and their partners would like to open up, the initial task is to help staff to feel more confident about tackling it. For some professionals it may be important to reframe their perception of sexual needs more broadly, as intimacy and closeness, rather than as simply sexual intercourse and penetration. Recognizing it is potentially an issue for all, however young, old or disabled a person, is a central principle. Fallowfield (1992) pleads for honesty at early stages of the illness about the possible effects of treatment on sexual function, fertility and libido, along with reassurance that the couple may well find a different but also satisfying relationship. Good prostheses or reconstructive surgery may be important at this stage. A factor that often stops professionals exploring any issue, not just sexual needs, is that they feel they may be expected to have the answers to all questions. Booth (1995) has shown that nurses were much more ready to open up discussion of sensitive topics if they felt supported by their manager and knew that practical help would be available if needed. So it is important that the professional knows the address and phone number of the local sexual health service or of an organization like SPOD, the national charity in the UK that has an advice service on sexual matters for people with disability, for those who need more specialist advice.

Monroe has some helpful suggestions for ways into this topic with the dying person and their partner (Monroe, 1993a). Putting this area forward as one that may have changed along with other areas gives the opportunity for the issue to be picked up or ignored – 'Cancer often brings big changes to all aspects of life. Has it brought any changes in your family relationships, your life as a couple, your ability to get close to one another physically?' This is a time when the multiple questions usually frowned upon by communications experts may actually have a purpose. By mentioning sexual life as one aspect among many the professional shows that they recognize it as a legitimate area for discussion. But not dwelling on it or singling it out gives an opportunity for it to be left aside or possibly returned to later. Enabling a couple to feel that they are not unusual in having questions or difficulties is a help. 'Many people have questions about the effects of their illness on the sexual side of life.' Here the professional has at least demonstrated that they are able to mention the topic and the couple may ask a question at a later meeting. Having books or pamphlets about illness and sexual issues in the literature stand at the out-patient clinic or on the ward also gives the message that this is an acceptable topic. Although it is probably helpful to make it clear at a meeting with both partners that sex can be discussed, it may well be that one of them will seek an individual interview. This could be where they are unable to talk about it together or where the patient has become very fearful of it. There are still those who fear that cancer particularly is contagious and could be spread by intercourse. Some carers feel that they should not have any concern for their own needs when a partner is dying and may avoid intimate contact, yet that dying partner may long for physical closeness. The professional may help to bring these anxieties out into the open by making general statements like 'Some people worry that the illness is catching and avoid close physical contact with those they love because of this'. As Monroe observes, a sense of humour, if used sensitively, can be an asset in such discussions.

5.2.4 Meeting the needs of children facing bereavement

The first requirement is that all those involved with children facing a death in the family realize that children cannot in practice be excluded from the situation. They will sense that adults are anxious, they may overhear conversations, a friend at school may pass on adult gossip. Lucy aged 11 was sitting watching television when the nurse from the hospice called to talk about finding extra help for Lucy's mother, who was caring for her dying sister Maxine. As Lucy's mother and the nurse stood at the door of the room where Lucy was sitting her mother said in a normal voice 'Of course, Lucy does not know that Maxine is dying'. Lucy did not turn round but her back stiffened and it was clear she had heard, but her mother did not seem to perceive this. Parents who want to 'protect' their children by saying nothing need to be helped to see how impossible it is to keep the knowledge from them. It may also be important for them to know, as described in the Setting the scene section, that quite young children can have a full understanding of the concept of death, and that knowledge of what is happening is seldom harmful in itself. Parents also need to reflect on the consequences if they tell older children and not younger children. When Anne was dying her three teenage daughters were told what was going to happen. One day going home from a visit to the hospice where she was an inpatient her 10-year-old son asked his stepfather if his mother was going to die. His stepfather lied and denied that she would. After her death this child had the most difficulties of all the children, some of which might be attributed to this exclusion. Once parents are ready to be more open the following guidelines can offer a framework for the discussion:

(a) Help parents to talk to their own children themselves.

They know the child best and the child is more likely to ask them questions in the course of everyday conversations, than to ask a relatively unknown professional. That is not to say that professionals may not have important roles. A key role is to support parents in being good parents even in this painful situation by assisting them in their efforts to prepare their children for the difficulties ahead. When it was clear that Jean's husband would not be returning home from hospital as planned and might die in the next few days, Jean decided she needed to prepare her three young daughters, twins of 9 and the other aged 7, for his death. Jean was judged to be of low intelligence and not very competent, so the ward staff were very relieved when she asked if a social worker would come and help her do this. The social worker had never met the family before. When she arrived Jean had asked her mother-in-law and a family friend to be present so that, as she put it, 'Everyone has someone to cuddle, because we are going to hear some sad news'. Making sure that each child was sitting on the knee of a familiar person, she proceeded to tell the little girls that their father would soon die. She did not use words the social worker would have used, or go about it in a professional way, but it was the way her children knew. The social worker was not required to say a word from start to finish. What she seemed to be needed for was to make it feel safe enough for Jean to do the work herself. Professionals may also have a part to play in answering some questions that the parents do not know the answer to. Parents may help their children to draw up a list of questions they would like to ask. For some parents it may be helpful to be able to rehearse how they will talk to their children and to discuss the conversation afterwards with a professional.

(b) Find out what the child already knows.

It is all too easy to assume that this particular child knows nothing about what is happening because they have never asked any questions or given a clue that they know. They may have developed an explanation for what is going on from the snippets that they have picked up which relates to reality, or they may have some completely false ideas. Using open questions – 'Mummy has been sick for a long time now. How do you think she is getting on?', 'What do you think made granddad ill?' – may give an opportunity to find out what these are. Demonstrating an interest in what the child thinks and feels may give them the courage to ask the question that is really bothering them, trivial though it may seem to adults. It may sometimes be helpful to say that some children worry that something they did has caused this terrible thing to happen. Magical thinking – feeling that our powerful, primitive angry thoughts and feelings have the potential to destroy others – can exist in both children and adults, but adults are usually more able to bring intellectual reasoning to their aid and overcome it. Hemmings (1994) gives an excellent example of a way of helping a child to deal with magical thinking, in that case a 4-year-old who thought that she had caused the cot death of her baby sister.

(c) Use simple language.

Children need to learn the language of death just like any other vocabulary. It is often difficult to use hard words like 'death' to adults and even more difficult when the person who must hear it is a vulnerable child who may feel very powerless. However, unless the child understands what is happening the situation will be even more overwhelming. So it is more essential to use the real, harsh words and to check that this child knows what death means or what happens at a funeral.

(d) Use play.

Children often express their thoughts and feelings through play rather than in face to face conversation. Using modelling materials, playing imaginative games or drawing they may focus on the situation facing them. The professional should not put their own interpretation on the material produced, but ask the child about it. Often a discussion around a drawing of their family will highlight their concerns or give an opportunity to build on their observations. Any specialist palliative care service should have available drawing and modelling materials. In an in-patient setting this should be in a welcoming area that makes it clear that this is specially for children to use. A small corner will do, with a box of toys, a small table and chair, and a pinboard so that drawings can be displayed if the child wishes. There are some commercially produced drawing books which offer children a framework of questions and observations to illustrate, e.g. the series by Marge Heegard (Heegard, 1991). However, it is equally satisfactory to staple some sheets of coloured paper together and suggest perhaps that the child make a scrapbook about hospitals or about their sick parent.

There are an increasing number of books for children of all ages that introduce the topic of death and dying. These range from picture books to be read by an adult with a young child to novels for teenagers. A specialist bookseller like Meditec in the UK may stock many of the titles. These may provide a useful way into the subject for parents with their children. Again every specialist palliative care service should have a small library of such books which can be lent to parents or to those caring for children facing bereavement.

(e) Recognize the individual relationship of the child with the dying person.

Each child in the family has their own special relationship with the person who is dying. It may be straightforward and loving, it may be tense and ambivalent or abusive. Whatever its quality it must be valued and the fact that an attachment exists recognized. Some children may wish to be very involved in the practical care of the dying person and this has certainly been shown to help the siblings of dying children make a better adjustment after the death (Lauer *et al.*, 1985). However, those who shun it should not be penalized or made to feel that they are less loved because they want to protect themselves from the pain of being too close. Adolescents particularly may choose to withdraw, as they wrestle with trying to balance their wish for independence with an event that inevitably draws them back into family life.

(f) Draw on the family and community support networks.

Professionals can encourage stunned and despairing parents to consider who in their local or family network may be able to offer extra support to the child or children. Adolescents may find it easier to talk to an aunt or uncle or old family friend who is not quite so closely affected as their own parents. Their peer group may actually offer more help than parents realize, particularly if there is someone in the group who has had a similar experience (Berman, Cragg and Kuenzig, 1988). Teachers in school or college can be an important source both of normality and support for a child, provided that they themselves are not afraid to mention the topic, and parents should be encouraged to give their child's school at least some idea of what is going on. The teacher may help the child or young person to decide how to share with classmates what is happening (*Information Exchange*, 1996). The specialist palliative care service may have a useful role to play in helping to ensure that local schools are able to be supportive and helpful to children facing bereavement by putting on study days for teachers or school nurses on child bereavement.

The needs of children who are acting as carers for a dying parent, often in single-parent families, are slowly being recognized. Jenny Frank carried out a sensitive study of young carers in Hampshire whose ages ranged from 3 to 17. Some of these families were already known to the health and welfare services, but the role of the children in caring had not always been recognized. She provides a useful checklist for helping to determine whether a child is a young carer, and principles and guidelines for working with young carers (Frank, 1995). Adolescents in single-parent families may have heavy demands for support placed on them by the dying person that they may resent or fear, but feel obliged to try to meet. For adolescents in split families the potential loss of one parent may reawaken the painful feelings from the time of the family break-up.

5.2.5 Family meetings

Carers have individual anxieties and needs which they may require one to one help with. However, in most situations when someone is dying it can be extremely helpful to meet the family or group of carers all together at least once, perhaps to plan a discharge, or to understand why problems are occurring. A family meeting may be a way of ensuring that children are included, whether they are 10 years old or the distressed adult children of Kissane *et al.*'s (1994) study. Monroe (1993a) and Smith and Regnard (1993) have provided some useful pointers towards making such meetings useful and relevant to both families and professionals.

Good planning is vital. If possible, working with another professional from a different background will help to ensure that all areas of potential difficulty are covered and may help to defuse any preconceptions that the family have about one particular group of professionals. The objectives for the meeting must be agreed by both professionals. Consider whether the dying person should be included in the meeting. If they are not they should certainly know that it is taking place, and there should be an agreement about how the proceedings are to be fed back to them. Be clear with the family about how much time is available for the discussion. 'The aim is to help them to solve their problems in a way that feels reasonably comfortable for them, not to sort everything out for them' (Monroe, 1993a). So it is important to know what the individual members of the family or group see as the problem, and to make sure that everyone there has their chance to have a say. Ask too what those who are not present might say, since they need to be taken into account as part of the system. To enable people to voice feelings or thoughts that they fear may be unacceptable, it may be helpful for the professional to normalize anything they suspect may be difficult by saying, for example 'Many people worry about how they will manage at home/ what they should say to the children/how they will pay for continuing care'.

As Smith and Regnard (1993) point out, families may be distressed but they do not automatically have problems when some one is dying, although it is not always possible to know this unless you ask them. Sometimes what is required is an endorsement of what they have done so far. They may think they are coping far less well than in fact they are. If there do seem to be difficulties, perhaps one member being scapegoated, competition over who most loves/is loved by the dying person, inability to agree on a way forward, then the professionals may be able to use the technique of positive reframing to unlock the situation. By acknowledging, for example, that the energy that is going into disagreements is a sign of how much everyone is concerned about the dying person and wants the best for them, and asking how we can use this energy for their benefit, those concerned may feel valued and safe enough to redirect that energy. The four very loving daughters of Anna who was dying of leukaemia could not sort out how to organize the help she needed. Each had a different but valuable contribution to make, arising from their own individual talents and circumstances. Each feared her sisters would criticize her for not doing as much or the same as they were. At the family meeting the nurse and the social worker present valued the different contributions – the older sister, a senior nurse, supported her mother on hospital visits, the youngest was hopeless at housework but could negotiate ably with the Department of Social Security, the second daughter was best at unobtrusive daily support as she lived near. This seemed to enable them to give up their fears and fantasies, and work together pooling their talents rather than competing.

If someone has reluctantly to change their behaviour or their views it is important to maintain their dignity. If the meeting is bringing together people with a legacy of bitterness from the past because of divorce or a family quarrel, then the professionals may need to recognize this at the start of the meeting and set some very clear boundaries: 'We know that things have been very difficult between you in the past. At this meeting it is important to discuss the situation as it is now reasonably calmly. If we find that people are becoming angry we shall take a cooling-off break.' Finally it is helpful if the professional team summarize what may have, been agreed and think with those there about how it will be conveyed to those who are not present but who are concerned in the situation.

5.2.6 The last days

There comes a time when it becomes clear that there is very little time left for this person, even to many of those who have been hoping against hope. Reimer and her colleagues (1991) have described this as the transition of 'fading away'. In their qualitative study of Canadian families of cancer patients they found this recognition came suddenly and was linked to irrecoverable loss – extreme weakness, inability to get around, loss of independence in personal care, loss of mental clarity. Families were then faced with the need to redefine their view of the world, confront the inevitability of death and tentatively begin to look to the future. Reimer *et al.* propose approaches for nurses which will be helpful for families at this time, although these approaches can equally well be applied by any member of the professional team. First, they suggest giving time and opportunities to talk about the loss that is coming and about losses that have happened on the way to this point – in other words, time to grieve. Recognize that different members of the family will take different amounts of time to assimilate the change and that each may react differently to it. While trying to ensure that the family have adequate resources to care, help to maintain the self-esteem of the dying person by still including them in family life and not denying them the responsibilities that they can take on. Annette, a 37-year-old single parent, was lying in bed in her living room two days before her death. She was thin and weak. Her two daughters, Jenny aged 9 and Mary aged 6, were playing quietly in a corner. As the visiting social worker and her mother were helping her to sit more upright in the bed, she stopped them and said to Jenny, 'Don't think that because I can't see you I don't know what you are doing'. She maintained a key element of her parental role – a firm and loving control of her children – long after she had had to give up physical care of them.

Once the approaching loss is acknowledged the families enter what Reimer and her colleagues describe as 'the neutral zone' where they are balancing a variety of conflicting pressures – carrying on with some normal routines but preparing for death, perhaps wanting the pain to end but feeling guilty about this, struggling with their own wishes and needs while trying to meet those of other family members. The professional role here is to provide a sounding board, to help people explore options and what is tolerable for them, and to validate and normalize their confused feelings – but beware of seeming to minimize what they are experiencing by too bland a reassurance that 'everyone feels like this at this time'. The uniqueness and particular power of this time for them is what needs to be valued.

Some families will begin to look to the future, even if only by revealing their concern about how they will meet the expenses of the funeral. Reimer and her colleagues recommend that professionals maintain a delicate balance here, not forcing the family to talk about difficult topics, but being alert for any hints and demonstrating that you are not frightened to talk of them. So saying 'have you ever thought at all what life might be like after he has died?' may offer a welcome opportunity to talk about some heavy anxiety. On the other hand, if it meets the response 'No, I can't bear to think of it' there is no need to press the point. They wisely remark that 'nurses must not expect that all families will achieve new beginnings. Some may never acknowledge endings and others will continue to struggle in the neutral zone. Nurses should not consider themselves or the families as having failed if new beginnings are not established. Transitions are processes, not achievements!' (Reimer *et al.*, 1991).

5.3 CONCLUSION

For the family or group of carers the death marks the beginning of another, possibly even more painful time – the time of bereavement. This will be the focus of the next chapter.

6 | Bereavement

6.1 SETTING THE SCENE

The process of bereavement starts as soon as someone acknowledges that this person they care about is going to die. This knowledge may be resisted, it may be only intermittently in consciousness but it begins to shape the expectations of the person who will survive and to change their assumptive world (Parkes, 1971). Indeed, this may be protective as well as painful. Parkes (1986) has shown that those who are prepared for a death, especially if the death is of an older person, are likely to have fewer problems in bereavement than those who experience sudden death. Although accurate predictions of life expectancy are notoriously difficult (Heyse-Moore and Johnson, 1987) it does usually becomes clear in the days before it happens that the actual death is approaching. This is probably most true for those with cancer, rather less so for those with cardiac disease or AIDS (Foley *et al.*, 1995). The experience of the survivor around the time of the death may affect their subsequent bereavement. One of the subjects the Issues in practice section will consider is what professionals need to take into consideration to make that event as least harmful as possible. However, it is important to look first at theoretical approaches to the process of bereavement and understand some of the debates about it. We are part of a particular society and are inevitably influenced by the ideas current in that society about bereavement. There has sometimes been a rather rigid approach on the part of professionals which sought to prescribe not only behaviour but feelings too. Here, as in relation to death, this book takes the neo-modern stance described by Walter (1994) and seeks to promote a flexible approach which respects the experience and wishes of bereaved individuals. Understanding what is influencing our thinking may help us to take such an approach.

6.1.1 The development of bereavement theory

There have been attempts to explain the experience of bereavement from a number of different theoretical perspectives. Bowlby's view (Bowlby, 1969) was that there was an underlying biological purpose in grief of trying to maintain group cohesion. Initially the bereaved person may try to regain proximity to the lost person through protest, searching and despair. These emotions may also prompt others in the bereaved person's social network to pay attention to and care for them. There have been attempts to examine physiological changes in bereavement and some evidence has been found that it may affect the neuroendocrine and immune systems (Kim and Jacobs, 1993; Irwin and Pike, 1993). Grief has been characterized as an illness (Engel, 1961) but this view has been much criticized by those who emphasize the crucial importance of the social context of grief and mourning practices. However, it is the psychology of grief that has had most theoretical attention.

Freud first developed a psychology of grief (Freud, 1917), but it was the work of Parkes in the 1960s and 1970s which gave a new impetus to the study of bereavement (Parkes, 1986). Drawing on Bowlby's theory of attachment and on his research with widows, he proposed a series of stages in the bereavement process. Initially there is a reaction of shock, numbness and disbelief, and this occurs to some degree even if the death is expected. As disbelief and numbness wane, they are succeeded by the pangs of grief. There are waves of overwhelming emotion which well up at any time. These may be of sadness, anger or guilt, or a mixture of them all. Parkes pointed out too the insecurity and fear which many bereaved people experience who face a new and threatening world without the person who made them feel loved and valued in the past. This has a physiological impact and may mean that a bereaved person will experience many of the feelings of severe anxiety – a knot in the pit of the stomach, an enhanced consciousness of their body, a restlessness, perhaps a searching for the dead person, and an inability to concentrate. A time of desolation and despair succeeds as the full realization that the dead person will not return strikes home. Gradually the bereaved person begins to re-involve themselves in life again and gains a new identity. From Freud Parkes took the idea of 'griefwork'. For Freud this was what needed to be done to detach the bereaved person from the dead person – a reality testing that helped them to realize that that person no longer exists. Parkes developed this in some detail. He suggested that it consisted of a preoccupation with thoughts of the dead person, a painful going over of the events surrounding the death and an attempt to make sense of the loss. He recognized that a number of different factors may determine the pace and the style of an individual's bereavement, and these will be considered later in the chapter.

Building on Parkes' work, Worden (1982) identified a series of tasks for the bereaved and this approach became extremely well-known. These were:

- Accepting the reality of the loss.
- Experiencing the pain of grief.
- Adjusting to a world in which the deceased is missing.
- Withdrawing emotional energy from the deceased and reinvesting it in another relationship.

Worden suggested that formulating the bereavement process as a series of tasks might give the bereaved person a sense of having something active to do, rather than having to passively endure a series of stages. Already by the late 1980s there were beginning to be challenges to the approaches developed by Parkes and Worden, and in the second edition of Worden's book, published in 1991 (Worden, 1991), he modified his final stage to:

- Finding an appropriate place for the deceased in the bereaved person's emotional life.

6.1.2 Challenges to accepted models

The challenges came from a number of directions. There was a concern that a rigid model had become current which did not necessarily fit the experience of all bereaved people. Wortman and Silver (1989) identified a number of 'myths' about coping with loss and tested these against evidence from research studies. They concluded that distress is not an inevitable part of the grief process nor is 'griefwork' essential, that some bereaved people, particularly those in western society who experience the death of a child, never find a meaning in the death and that the expectation that all bereaved people will recover after a relatively short time is not borne out by the studies. They suggested from their review of bereavement research that there might in fact be three different patterns of response to the death of a loved one:

- Moving from high distress to low distress over time – the pattern identified by Parkes.
- Never experiencing high distress.
- Continuing in high distress for years.

Although some of their interpretations of the work of others can be criticized, they did disturb what had become a rather complacent acceptance of existing models.

Walter puts forward the idea that the reason for the popularity of the approaches of Parkes and Worden were twofold (Walter, 1994). First, those who most enthusiastically took up the ideas were practitioners in the field of bereavement counselling or palliative care. Those who came to ask for their help were most likely to be following the first or third pattern identified by Wortman and Silver. They seldom saw the second group. Secondly, work with the first group was satisfying as they improved over time. It was preferable to normalize that response as it gave both the worker and the bereaved person hope. Just as the widespread acceptance of the ideas of Elisabeth Kuebler-Ross may well have been because they helped professionals to contain their sense of chaos and despair in the face of death, so too a model of bereavement which suggests that the outcome of this painful process is acceptance and detachment from the deceased, gave a feeling of order and relief to those alongside the bereaved. Similarly this may again have led to an over-simplification of the original ideas as they seeped into practice.

The criticism was taken further by Margaret Stroebe in her review of the griefwork hypothesis (Stroebe, 1992–93). She demonstrated the difficulty of distinguishing between griefwork and obsessive rumination, which is widely agreed to be unhelpful, and showed that there was very little research evidence for the value of griefwork, defined as a strategy of attending to and confronting loss, except in situations of pathological grief where there was marked avoidance or excessive concentration on grief.

A second area of concern was the applicability of the models to non-western cultures. Bereavement research and the popular autobiographical accounts of bereavement such as C.S. Lewis's *A Grief Observed* (1961) emerged from North America and Northern Europe for the most part. Anthropologists had made many studies of the rituals surrounding death and bereavement in other cultures, but these had not been incorporated into the theoretical thinking underpinning palliative and bereavement care. Eisenbruch (1984) was one of the first to question the universality of grief and ask whether states of grief occur in the same sequence and at the same rate in all cultures, but his work was not widely known. Stroebe (1992–93) drew attention to work by Wikan comparing emotional experience and the approach to bereavement in two Muslim societies, Bali and Egypt. In Bali the bereaved were helped by others to avoid suffering through distraction, whereas in Egypt they were encouraged to dwell on their loss. The rationale for each approach was the same. Bereavement was recognized as a risk to health and the different styles in each society were designed to reduce that risk. Walter (1996) has pointed out that many cultures such as the Japanese actively include ancestors in the everyday life of the family and seek to maintain the presence of the deceased rather than detach from it, while others like the Balinese and the English do not.

In fact the degree to which grief is socially constructed had taken second place in the accepted models, which gave greater prominence to the psychological aspects of grief. The recognition of the differences between cultures in the expression of grief and of mourning customs has led to a greater appreciation of the differences within countries like the UK. The rituals surrounding a death in the Outer Isles of Scotland, where men may follow the coffin and women visit the grave after the funeral, are very different from a funeral in Southampton and different again from the way a family of West Indian origin celebrates a death in Brixton. As Rosenblatt (1993) observes 'Culture is such a crucial part of the context of bereavement that it is often impossible to separate an individual's grief from culturally required mourning... Presumably what people do in grieving feels real to them, and their expressions of grief in accord with cultural rules validate the rules and become part of the context of grief for others'.

Another aspect of bereavement theory where it was recognized that a more critical approach was required was in relation to differences between men and women. There has been considerable debate about whether men and women grieve differently – indeed it is a very common topic in bereavement support groups among bereaved people themselves. Certainly there is evidence that while death rates are higher in general for the bereaved in the first two years after the death across all cultures and socioeconomic groups, the rates are highest for widowers (Stroebe and Stroebe, 1993). There is a marked increase in suicide in the first week after bereavement, greatest for men, and the stress of bereavement is probably linked to the higher incidence of death from heart diseases in all bereaved compared with the non-bereaved. However, it can be argued that the differences found in the ways men and women respond to the loss of a loved one relate to the different expectations and roles of men and women in particular societies rather than to any biological difference. In western society men may often link to social support through female partners and may be less adept at seeking social support after their deaths. Fish (1986) found that mothers of children who die experience more guilt and anger than the fathers. However, it is unclear what role the father's greater opportunities of distraction through work may play in this. There is a need for more studies to examine the effect of male unemployment and of women's greater participation in the labour market on this finding (Hartley, 1996).

Some of the differences attributed to men and women in grief may in fact be due to bias in some of the research studies. Most bereavement research has concentrated on the loss of a heterosexual partner and women agree to participate more readily than men. So the applicability of models of bereavement derived mostly from studies of the experience of women who have lost male partners may be limited. Moreover, Stroebe and Stroebe (1993) found in a longitudinal study of younger widows and widowers in Germany that the widows approached who agreed to partic-ipate were more depressed than those who refused, whereas the widowers who participated were less distressed than those who refused. They suggest that this is because men in German society find it more difficult to break down and cry than women. The most distressed men would therefore be reluctant to expose themselves to a possibly emotional interview with a bereavement researcher. It is more acceptable for women to seek support and express strong emotion.

6.1.3 New approaches to bereavement theory

Out of these challenges have come new theoretical views of bereavement which attempt to incorporate the criticisms and build models more related to the complex experience of different bereaved people. Stroebe (1994) has proposed the Dual Process Model to take account of Wortman and Silver's criticism that there are three predominant patterns of grief, not one, and the research findings that failure to express emotion did not necessarily result in poor outcome in bereavement. She suggests that bereaved people are working on two different aspects of their situation, which she calls loss-orientation and restoration-orientation. When they are focusing on loss-orientation they are preoccupied with thoughts of the dead person, crying over the death, visiting the grave. When they are focusing on restoration-orientation they are distracting themselves from painful thoughts by work or play, involving themselves in new experiences. Most bereaved people oscillate between these two processes in a effort to protect themselves from the exhausting physiological consequences of too much energy being focused on suppression or on facing pain. In the early days of bereavement the concentration is more likely to be on the loss, as time goes on more on the restoration. Different individuals will have different balances between the two, depending on the circumstances of the loss, their personality and their cultural background. This model also addresses some of the differences between men and women. Men have been found to rely on problem-focused strategies of coping in western society, so may tend to use the restoration-orientation mode more. Women more frequently use emotion-focused strategies so may engage more with loss-orientation. Stroebe does agree that a concentration on one orientation to the exclusion of the other signifies pathology. Prolonged preoccupation with the loss would equate to chronic grief, persistent suppression with delayed or inhibited grief.

Walter draws on his own experience of bereavement to develop a model which emphasizes the importance of constructing a biography of the dead person which helps the bereaved to integrate the memory of the dead into their on-going lives (Walter, 1996). He suggests that in western society where the influence of tradition has waned, where geographical and social mobility means that neighbours or work colleagues may have little knowledge of an elderly person who has died, where a death in hospital may have excluded the bereaved person from much of what happened round the death, a new process is needed to achieve the resolution of Worden's fourth task – finding an appropriate place for the deceased in the bereaved person's emotional life (Worden, 1991). 'The process by which this is achieved is principally conversation with others who knew the deceased.' (Walter, 1996). This means a shift from the expression of feelings about the loss, which he asserts bereavement counsellors have concentrated on, to an emphasis on talking about the dead person with those who knew them or with those who will listen. Other biographical material such as letters of condolence or writings by the dead person may help to complete the picture. The objective is to retain the dead person and take them forward into the new life of the bereaved person, but in a different way from the past. This does not sound so very different from the process of internalization of the lost object described by Freud and his followers (Middleton *et al.*, 1993). Evidence from Silverman and Worden's prospective study of bereaved children in Massachusetts supports Walter's view that retaining the dead person is important. By the end of the first year of their bereavement 71% of the children were still thinking of their dead parent several times a week and 74% had kept something belonging to that person (Silverman and Worden, 1993). Walter acknowledges that his model requires empirical testing and that it may be a model more of a man's way through grief than woman's. The implications of these new theoretical approaches for practice will be discussed in the Issues in practice section.

6.1.4 What influences the grief process?

Whatever the theoretical model of grief, it is clear from a number of research studies (Parkes, 1990) that a number of factors may intensify, reduce or lengthen the impact of the bereavement. One has already been mentioned – preparation for the death tends to reduce the incidence of problems in bereavement. Over-long preparation can however nullify this. One study (Gerber *et al.*, 1975) found that those who have nursed someone for over six months may have more difficulties, perhaps because this has caused them to lose contact with the social supports that can act as buffer, perhaps because the health of an elderly carer may have deteriorated under the stress of caring. Contrariwise, those who experience a sudden death are more likely to have difficulties. Feelings of shock and disbelief may last much longer as the sudden change from normal everyday life is so hard to take in. An added factor may be that sudden death may be associated with violence (murder or suicide) or with an accident where someone may be to blame. In these circumstances too the bereaved may experience post-traumatic stress disorder with high anxiety, flashbacks and nightmares in addition to the bereavement.

There has been considerable debate about the concept of anticipatory grief. Does it exist? What are its characteristics? In her review of research on the concept of anticipatory grief Evans (1994) points out the confusion in this area. There is a fundamental difference between 'anticipatory grief' and the grief following the actual death. What carers, family and friends are experiencing before the death is not just the anticipation of the terminal event, but also all the losses that the illness may bring. In contrast to grief after the event, the sadness felt before the event may increase in intensity as the death approaches, rather than diminish, a common pattern after a death. Evans pleads for a re-naming of the experience before the death – preferring to call it the 'terminal response' – to avoid muddled thinking.

Age at bereavement can be a factor. In western society loss of a partner at a young age carries more of a risk for women than at an older age, perhaps because it is no longer expected that young people will die. Older widowers are more at risk (Young, Benjamin and Wallis, 1963). Brown and Harris in their study of factors that influence the development of depression in women found that women whose mother had died when they were under the age of 11 were more likely to develop depression. This was especially found for women who had not received good care after their mother's death (Brown and Harris, 1978).

Parkes and Weiss (1983) found that those with an ambivalent relationship with the dead person were more likely to have problems. This may be because death has not only robbed them of the person who was significant to them but also robbed them of the chance to put right what went wrong. Those with a sense of a good relationship carry that helpfully into bereavement. When Nigel, a senior naval officer, knew he was within a few days of death he asked the nurses to call his wife in, and he thanked her for being such a good wife and taking so much responsibility for the family when he was overseas. She missed him deeply in her bereavement, but the memory of this conversation was a great support to her. A dependent relationship between the dead person and the bereaved person tends also to slow down the resolution of grief – no matter which appeared the most dependent. Personality must influence the grief process. Lund and colleagues found that the elderly in their sample who had poor self-esteem before the death were more likely to be coping worse than the rest two years after the bereavement (Lund *et al.*, 1985–86).

Stigmatized deaths too increase the pain for the bereaved. Suicide may be associated with high levels of anger or guilt and those bereaved by suicide show in their turn a higher tendency to commit suicide. This may be linked either to the manner of the bereavement, or to pre-existing shared family problems which influenced the first suicide such as heavy drinking or depression.

AIDS is a disease which appeared first in the stigmatized groups of male homosexuals and drug users in North America and Europe.

Homosexual partners of those who have died from AIDS may be excluded from family funerals and if they are also infected may face their own death from the same disease in the near future (Sanders, 1993).

Lack of social support has been identified as a predictor of poor outcome in the first year of bereavement but social support is a complex phenomenon. As Stylianos and Vachon observe in their review of the role of social support in bereavement, 'Social support is a transactional process requiring, for its optimal provision, a fit among the donor, the recipient and the particular circumstances' (Stylianos and Vachon, 1993). A volunteer from a Bereavement Support Service was regularly visiting a distressed elderly widower. He did not seem to be becoming any less distressed. In time the volunteer discovered that the man was also being visited by two other volunteer services, one connected with the church, another with a charity. For him the fit was not the right one and he may even have derived some secondary gain from the number of visitors he was having, which would be jeopardized if he showed improvement in his spirits. Social support may include giving information, practical assistance, feedback on the views or behaviour of the bereaved person, or emotional support. As we saw in Chapter 5 it can have negative as well as positive aspects. Maddison and Walker (1967) found that those who perceived their family as unhelpful were likely to have a poor outcome in bereavement. Parkes sums up: 'secure people whose experience of life has lead to a reasonable trust in themselves and others will cope well with anticipated bereavements, provided they are well supported by a family who respects their need to grieve. However, multiple or unexpected and untimely losses of people on whom one depends or who depended on the survivor can overwhelm the most secure person and lack of security and support can undermine a person's capacity to cope with all types of bereavement' (Parkes, 1990)

6.1.5 Pathological grief – does it exist?

The factors listed above have been described as risk factors in that they may increase vulnerability to poor mental and physical health and produce poor coping compared with others. However, there are considerable difficulties in developing a definition of pathological grief (Middleton et al., 1993). The influence of culturally determined mourning practices, pre-existing personality disorder, the overlap with the syndromes of anxiety or depression are all difficult to separate out from the grief process. Thus it may be more appropriate to describe grief as a risk factor for developing anxiety or depression rather than the other way round. Similarly it may be that a complicated grief reaction is a sign of a pre-existing personality disorder. As we have seen the models of grief like Stroebe's Dual Process Model can accommodate a failure to express much overt

grief, which might using another model be described as absent or inhibited grief. The meaning of the loss – a very individual thing – is central
(Wortman, Silver and Kessler, 1993). As account is taken of the many
different factors that will influence this individual bereaved person's grief
'It is less and less possible to think that pathological grief will become a
unitary concept. Instead, future research will likely adopt a multidimen-
sional framework in conceptualising what may appear to be similar
consequences, or pathologies, but which derive from very different sources
and develop along very different paths' (Middleton *et al.*, 1993). The
consequences of this understanding for those offering bereavement
support services will be considered in the Issues in practice section.

6.1.6 Effective intervention

Surveys of palliative care bereavement services in the UK (Payne and
Relf, 1994; Wilkes, 1993) have shown that the most common types of
service offered to bereaved people are individual visits, group sessions
which range from therapeutic groupwork to social activities and telephone
contact. A smaller number of services send cards on the anniversary of
the death or arranged memorial services commemorating all those who
have died over a particular period. A few referred the bereaved to a
community bereavement support service like Cruse. Volunteers who have
had varying lengths of training carry out most of the interventions organized and supported mainly by social workers or nurses, although
professionals may be involved in assessment or in the more difficult situations. There have been a number of attempts to evaluate the different
types of intervention. An early study by Cameron and Parkes (1983)
seemed to suggest that the care offered by a hospice before the death and
one or two visits supplemented by telephone counselling after the death
combined to improve the outcome for those who received it, but this was
not borne out by a later larger study. Individual bereavement counselling
has been shown to be most effective for those assessed as at risk, particularly where the bereaved perceive their families as unhelpful (Raphael,
1983), but to be of little benefit for unselected groups (Parkes, 1990). Relf
(1997) found that the use of trained bereavement volunteers reduced the
use of GP services by her sample when compared with the control group.
Lieberman has reviewed research on the efficacy of self-help groups for
the bereaved which may or may not have a degree of professional help.
He found some basis for suggesting that generally such groups are helpful,
but nothing more precise than that (Lieberman, 1993). There has only
been evaluation of sending anniversary cards or holding memorial services
on a very small scale (Hutchinson, 1995; Foulstone, 1993). These findings
have implications for those developing bereavement services which will
be discussed in the Issues in practice section.

6.2 ISSUES IN PRACTICE

6.2.1 Around the time of death

Since the time around the death is remembered in considerable detail by many bereaved people services must be provided at that time which are as sensitive as possible to the needs of those who will survive, although if there is a conflict the needs of the dying person must have a high priority. Marianne, a divorced woman, was dying in a hospice. Her ex-husband was deeply distressed at her condition despite having another partner, and had been visiting her regularly. He wanted to be kept closely informed and to be there when she was dying. She confessed to the staff that she was finding his visits increasingly burdensome and it was agreed that he should be asked to stop visiting, although it was recognized that this would very much upset him and might make his bereavement more difficult. He would be offered bereavement support after her death.

The time of death poses different problems depending on where the death takes place. In an institutional setting you are in charge and can shape the experience to a degree, hopefully in conformity with the wishes of the dying person and their carers, but there are constraints because of the environment and the demands of other patients or residents. At home you are an adviser, although potentially a powerful one. Since carers are less likely to be present at the death if it occurs in hospital rather than in a hospice or at home (Lunt *et al.*, 1985) and there is evidence that many carers who were not there wished to be (Hampe, 1975; Sykes, Pearson and Chell, 1992), the first challenge is to ensure that those who wish to be there are there, but that those who wish to stay away can do so without fear of criticism. This means tackling the issue of whether the carer wishes to be called in at any time of the day or night in the event of deterioration on admission of any patient with life-threatening illness, even if death is not expected this admission. Presenting the choices in an even-handed way should help the carer not to feel pressurized one way or another – 'We are not necessarily expecting that he will get worse, but if it did happen would you prefer to be told straight away, even in the middle of the night, or to wait until morning? Some people prefer to wait, others want to know straight away'. However, their choice should be reviewed as the admission progresses in case it changes. Help the key carer to think what the wishes of those not present might be. Ask particularly about those who may be less able to speak for themselves – the elderly confused, young children or those with learning disabilities – and how they will say their goodbyes. Having a room to which carers can retreat in privacy is a bonus, but even showing them the quietest corner of the hospital canteen gives the message of concern for their distress and exhaustion.

Once someone has died different carers want to spend different amounts of time with the body and there is no 'right' amount of time. In a hospital setting there may be constraints because of pressure or staff shortages. If the body does have to be moved before the carers have finished, they should have time to prepare for this. Some carers, perhaps particularly those who have been involved in physical care of the dead person, may appreciate being asked if they would like to help wash and prepare the body. It is important not to ignore the feelings of any other patients in the ward or residential setting at the time of the death. They may have had a relationship with the dead person which extended over many years of visits to the same out-patients' clinics or residence in a home. They may not know them at all, but may be thinking about their own approaching death and how it may be handled. Research studies (Honeybun, Johnston and Tookman, 1992) in hospices have shown that patients are reassured by the way staff deal with it, rather than frightened by coming so close to death. So it is important to make sure that patients in the area or residents of the home know that the person has died and this is probably best done on an individual basis, to give an opportunity for any very personal questions to be asked.

In many hospices when carers return the following day to collect the death certificate and the dead person's belongings they will be given an opportunity to meet the primary nurse or doctor, and talk as they feel the need about any issues around the death. In hospitals this may be more difficult to arrange and the handover is usually carried out by an administrative officer, but carers will appreciate being taken over to the office by a member of staff who knew the dead person and the opportunity for discussion that that allows.

At home it is also useful to talk about the time of death before it is imminent, to allay any fears and ensure that the level of support that the carer requires is available if at all possible. Again this should be reviewed regularly as time goes on in case of any change. Since death at home is so much less frequent today, few carers even of middle age will have any previous experience of this. They may be unaware that they can take their time over saying goodbye, that the doctor does not have to be called in the middle of the night if he has been visiting the patient recently, that other relatives or friends may be called to make their farewells before the funeral director removes the body. It may be particularly important for the body not to be spirited away too quickly so that children can say good bye when they return home from school. In one residential home where an elderly couple were resident, the husband died. The staff left his body in their bedroom for 24 hours so that his confused wife could go in and out and over time experience that he was dead. They were convinced that this helped her to accept his death with relatively few repeated questions.

6.2.2 Assessing who is at risk in bereavement

How are we to take account of the developments in bereavement theory in practice? We have seen in Setting the scene how a wider range of behaviour and feelings in bereavement are being recognized as being 'normal', and that any assessment for deciding whether someone is at risk must take into account a wide range of factors about that individual's culture, personality and life experience. This means that there is no simple answer to the question of who is at risk. Yet there is an imperative to make best use of the scarce resources available in any service for bereavement care and to ensure that those who need extra help receive it. Payne and Relf (1994), in their survey of palliative care bereavement services, found that only 25% of their sample were using a risk index, usually based on Parkes' work on the determinants of grief (1986). As they point out, studies of its reliability have shown it to be predictive of outcome at three months, but not at other times in the bereavement. Parkes' own work did show nurses' gut feeling to be a good predictor of problems and there is a case for setting more value on clinical skills, but trying to be more systematic and monitoring outcomes. It may be more realistic for those working in the community to rely more on gut feeling since they usually have more time with the carer and more rounded information about the situation, although the greater closeness of the relationship may mean that it is more difficult for the nurse to detach herself and make an objective assessment. Clinical supervision and monitoring therefore become all the more important. For those working in hospital, and even in hospices where much shorter admissions are becoming the norm and contact with carers less, the use of an index of the risk factors identified in Setting the scene is most appropriate to identify those who are most likely to need individual support. Parkes points out that different settings and different populations of bereaved people require an adjustment of the risk index to take account of this. Since death is usually expected to some degree in a hospice a risk index there would need to put less weight on mode of death than one in an accident and emergency department (Parkes, 1990).

6.2.3 Providing services for bereaved people

Given that risk assessment is rather a blunt instrument for determining who will have particular difficulty and that bereavement is a painful time for the majority of those who have lost someone close to them, whether or not they are particularly at risk, there is an argument for having a range of different types of service available for bereaved people. The individual can then select what they feel to be appropriate. Some may reject the offer of one-to-one support after the death but welcome a telephone contact some weeks later which gives an opportunity to make another assessment of risk. Some will be helped by clear written information. Preparing a leaflet giving an outline of common feelings in bereavement and a list of local and national support groups may be all the professional help they need. Some will reject any help from the palliative care service because of its associations and will prefer a community service. It does make good sense for the bereavement service which is part of a specialist palliative care service to build good links with local voluntary bereavement support groups or other specialist services in the area, so that they can share expertise and training opportunities.

A general invitation to meet others in a similar situation at regular meetings at a hospice will be taken up by some. If this group is a closed group it will usually be clear at the start how many times it will meet. While the timing may not be right for every member there will be an opportunity for individual help for any identified as in need. If the group is an open group which people can join at any time attention has to be paid to enabling members of the group to leave the group when they have less need of support, so that there may be room for others at an earlier point in their grief to join. One hospice solved this problem by running a programme of 12 monthly meetings with speakers and time for socializing which a bereaved person could join at any point and knew that they would have to leave once they had attended all 12 in the cycle (Celia Cooke, personal communication).

Volunteers can play a large part in a bereavement support service undertaking one-to-one support and participating in providing telephone calls and group sessions. But they will only be effective and safe if they are properly selected, trained and supported. This does not mean that they have to become mini-professionals, but it should ensure that they are prepared for the common problems that they will meet and can look after themselves and the bereaved whom they wish to help. Those setting up the service need to be clear. Is the aim to have bereavement befrienders whose main task will be to support any suffering bereaved person through the normal course of their grief by sensitive listening and empathetic support or is it to have bereavement counsellors (with all that implies about length of training) working with those whose grief is more problematic? Earnshaw-Smith and Yorkstone have produced a good guide to setting up and running a volunteer bereavement service (Earnshaw-Smith and Yorkstone, 1986), and the National Association of Bereavement Services can provide advice and information.

6.2.4 Meeting the needs of vulnerable groups

Making sure that less powerful members of society have their needs met in bereavement is an important preventive role for professionals in palliative care. Young children, the frail or confused elderly person or some one with learning disabilities may be excluded from open discussions about what is happening in a well-meaning attempt to protect them. Yet their lifestyle may be radically changed by the death. Oswin (1993) gives painful examples of failures to tell people with learning disabilities about the death of a parent, leaving them worrying about their absence or resentful that they were not included. Those whose understanding may be limited need more help not less. In Chapter 5 we considered some principles to underpin work with children facing bereavement, and these principles are just as valid once the death has occurred and can be adapted for work with other vulnerable groups.

Following the greater emphasis on openness at this time there has been considerable development of bereavement services geared particularly to children's needs. Some of this has been on an individual basis using drawing and play to help children express their feelings and questions (Hemmings, 1994). Games have been developed for this purpose. One, a board game, *All About Me*, has a series of cards with questions which child and worker pick up as they land on a board square (Barnardo's, 1992). The worker can tailor the cards to the needs of this particular child. Since the worker is also answering questions the child is not too exposed. Others have worked with family groups (Firth and Anderson, 1994) and Hildebrand describes a case with good examples of ways of recognizing childrens' anxieties or opening up dialogue (Hildebrand, 1989).

However, the most development has occurred in groups for bereaved children. These have been developed by a number of different organizations – hospices, child guidance clinics, voluntary groups – and in a variety of formats. A popular arrangement is to invite up to 10 children to come for four or five hours, during which they may play games, work on a family tree or paint and draw on topics related to their bereavement. Familiar, comforting food such as crisps, pizzas and soft drinks are a feature of the session. There should be at least one member of staff to two children and art therapists are often asked to participate (Baulkwill and Wood, 1994; Burroughs *et al.*, 1992). Some groups spread similar activity over several shorter sessions over a period of weeks, and may include outings to graveyards and relaxation sessions (Pennells and Kitchener, 1990). A particularly creative approach to running such groups has used bereaved adolescents as helpers at a group for younger bereaved children with benefit to both parties (Ann Ball, personal communication).

One of the most elaborate programmes for bereaved children is the Winston's Wish programme developed in Gloucestershire by Julie Stokes and her colleagues. This started initially as a weekend camp for bereaved children with volunteer and professional helpers where they participate in games and rituals such as lighting a candle for the dead person and sending off a balloon with the name of the person on it. An important session is 'Doctor's Questions' where children work with a helper to produce a question that concerns them about the illness or death of the person they were close to. These are then anonymized and the doctor answers them in front of the whole group (Thompson, 1996). The Winstons' Wish programme has now extended into work in schools with groups of bereaved children. In all these different types of group careful planning involving all who will be helping is vital. Visits to parents or carers and children before the group, to give the invitation and to explain what will happen, are an important contributor to making both feel that participation will be safe and useful.

There has been much less concentration on elderly people with confusion who are bereaved. However, some principles and practice are emerging. First and foremost it is an ethical issue. A confused person has a right to know something so important about someone close to them. Then too there is much more appreciation now of the extent to which those with Alzheimer's disease may be aware of what is happening, even if that understanding is clouded or partial. Behaviour may show this even if words do not. It is important to talk with close relatives in some detail about how they will give the news. Reassuring the confused person that the dead person is at peace and safe may help to minimize any anxiety reaction (Mackay, 1993). Participation in the funeral will assist in making the loss more real. A family member or friend who is not too distressed can usefully take responsibility for looking after the confused person during the ceremony to enable others to be free to grieve. Benbow and Quinn (1990) demonstrate that a planned programme of visits to the grave by the confused person, with a helper who can use the opportunity to talk about the death, can promote comprehension. As always the approach has to be individual, taking into account the degree of dementia and keeping communication simple and clear. Every detail of the death does not have to be shared but any questions should have a truthful response. A similar approach may be taken with those with learning disabilities.

Other groups who may have particular difficulty in bereavement are those experiencing stigmatized deaths such as suicide, or those whose mourning may be hidden or ignored. The death of a partner in a gay relationship may be an example here. The Lesbian and Gay Bereavement project in London has a telephone helpline. Such services are particularly useful for those who are not part of a supportive gay community. Contact with others in the same situation can be supportive and reassuring. Group sessions especially for the relatives or close friends of those who commit suicide give opportunities to talk about any feelings of pain, shame or anger and show that your experience is not unique. These may be set up by mental health services.

6.2.5 Working with difficult problems in bereavement

The majority of people go through the bereavement process with help
from only friends and family, a minority welcome support from services
at painful times in their progress, some need more specialist help. A few
become chronic grievers. If you are faced with someone whose grief is
unusually intense and unusually long-lasting, taking into account all the
factors which have broadened our view of normal grief, then a careful
assessment is needed. Is it self-punitive, due to guilt about some aspect
of the loss? Is it from a sense of misplaced loyalty, a fear that others will
think you did not really love the dead person if you stop grieving? A man
at a bereavement group for men, all about six months bereaved, asked
other group members with great intensity if they found that they sometimes didn't think of their dead wife for perhaps half an hour at a time.
They reassured him that this was the same for them but they saw it as
normal and part of having, however regretfully, to move on in life. This
seemed to give him permission to move on and he was in fact the first of
the group to re-marry.

Is it fear of the future that maintains the person in grief? Here a
programme which step by step supports the bereaved person in developing a new identity can be helpful. This may be by a trusted helper
setting them goals which they should achieve by the next meeting. Mary's
husband had accompanied her everywhere. After his death she was too
frightened to go out and only managed to buy food by taking a taxi to
the corner shop at the end of the road. A volunteer won her trust and
Mary agreed to walk to the shop if she came with her. By the end of the
contact three months later Mary was going alone on the bus to meet the
volunteer at the supermarket in town and was attending a luncheon club.

Techniques like writing a letter to the dead person or imaging they are
sitting in an empty chair and talking to them may be useful with those
who are torturing themselves with guilt or anger. These should be used
as part of a planned piece of work with the bereaved person. Even if they
do not want to show you the letter or talk in front of you, it is important
to give them an opportunity to discuss with you how it went and what
any outcome has been. For those who have been excluded from a death
or cannot make it real because they have not seen the body, developing
a series of rituals with them that help them to take a formal good-bye of
the dead person can be helpful. Behaviour therapy for unduly prolonged
and profound grief has been used successfully by Ramsay (1977) and
Mawson et al. (1981), but this should only be attempted with input from
the psychiatric services.

We have seen in Setting the scene that bereaved people may be at risk
of committing suicide. It is therefore important to take seriously any hints
given or threats made. Parkes recommends asking 'Has it been so bad

that you thought of taking your own life?' if you are worried (Parkes, 1982). This will not put the idea into the person's head, since most unhappy people think of suicide, if only to dismiss it. If it becomes clear to you that there is a real risk of it happening, it is your responsibility to inform the person's GP, even if they do not wish you to do so. This is one occasion on which it is permissible to break the confidential relationship. Most bereaved people will understand your position. Some may be relieved to have the help brought to them. Parkes reminds us that, if they agree, staying in touch with the person over the crisis may be particularly important, even if other services have become involved.

If a bereaved person you have been working with closely commits suicide you may have in some degree similar feelings and questions to those experienced by family members in this situation. This is awful. What could I have done to prevent it? How could he/she do this to me? Will others blame me? You should be offered opportunities to make sense of what has happened and to examine what you have been responsible for, and what was the responsibility of others, even the responsibility of the person who has committed suicide. It is important to learn from what has happened and to accept what is properly yours – but it is equally important not to take responsibility for elements in the situation which you could not have changed. This is a time when the support of the team or your manager is particularly needed and you should not be afraid to ask for this.

6.3 CONCLUSION

In our efforts to understand bereavement and target resources effectively sometimes we 'see a symptom and miss the wound' (Karl, 1987). Working with bereaved people we are often in contact with overwhelming emotional pain. But we need to recognize their strengths too. Payne and Relf (1994) point out that we have often been more preoccupied with pathology than with resilience. The more we work with bereaved people the more we can appreciate the very different paths along which they move into the future.

7 | Working in palliative care

7.1 SETTING THE SCENE

So far in this book, the dying person, carers and family have been centre stage. We now shift to concentrating more on the professionals working in palliative care. Unless that work experience is reasonably satisfying and stimulating most of the time, it is unlikely that the outcomes for dying people and their carers will be acceptable or in tune with the principles of palliative care. This section will look at stresses for staff, teamwork in palliative care and advocacy. Team building, multiprofessional learning, staff support systems and handling conflict in teams will be the topics in Issues in practice.

7.1.1 Sources of stress for staff caring for people who are dying

There are now a large number of studies looking at what causes stress for those working with dying people and, as we shall see, some interesting differences have emerged between those who work in specialist settings and those who work in general settings. A cautionary note – the majority of studies have been carried out with women participants, most frequently nurses. So it is unclear how applicable the research findings are to the experience of male staff or other professions. In addition there has been rather little consideration of the effect of cultural differences on staff stress in palliative care. Most of the studies have been carried out in the USA and the UK and differences in, for example, the organization and funding of health and social care and levels of religious affiliation and commitment mean that work in one society may only have limited relevance for the other. A further factor to take into account is the changing nature of stress in specialist settings as services move from the pioneer phase to a greater integration in general health and social care systems. Of course this might also have an impact on the stress felt by those caring for dying people in general settings in two ways. As the principles and practices of specialist palliative care become included in basic professional education and therefore more widespread in general settings, professionals working there may feel better prepared to deal with any problems. They may also be more likely to be able to call on the skills of a specialist hospital or community support team.

Vachon, a major contributor to research in this area, has proposed a model of occupational stress which describes it as the result of a dynamic interaction between the person holding a particular job and the environment in which he or she is employed. 'Job stress results when the individual's supplies and resources do not mesh with the demands of the work environment. (Vachon, 1995). From research studies she identifies a number of different elements (Figure 7.1) which are key in this interaction.

We have seen in Chapter 1 that the personal values, qualities and past experience that professionals bring to their work are bound to shape the care that they offer. Studies have shown that those in specialist settings who are older and have been longer in the job perceive less stress (Dunne

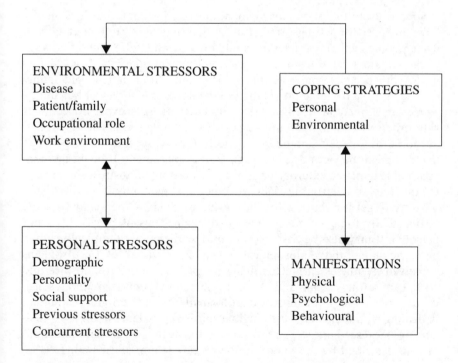

Figure 7.1 Model of occupational stress. Redrawn with permission from Vachon, M.L.S. (1995) Staff stress in hospice/palliative care: a review. *Palliative Medicine,* **9**(2), 91–122.

and Jenkins, 1991). Social support is a key factor, but as we have seen in relation to carers in Chapter 5 it can cut both ways – it can be a buffer or a stress in itself. Vachon (1995) reports that being married and having children was associated with more job satisfaction in Sweden but having dependants was associated with more stress in the USA. This might well be due in its turn to the greater support for parents and carers in the Swedish welfare system. Religious affiliation frequently brings with it a social support system and this may make it hard to tease out whether religious faith or the support system have contributed to the significance of this factor. Wilkinson found that nurses who had a religious affiliation were less likely to use blocking tactics in communicating with patients (Wilkinson, 1991). Similarly stressful life events may strengthen the worker if they contribute to emotional maturity and a well-worked out philosophy of life, but add to work stress if they are unresolved. A qualitative study by Pitcher of the effect of a personal bereavement on hospice nurses demonstrates the double edge of the experience – giving the nurses at the same time more understanding of carers but making it harder to face the patients who might be suffering from the same illness as their own relative (Pitcher, 1996).

Stresses from the work environment are rated as more burdensome by those in specialist settings than stresses that may arise from contact with dying people or their carers. One study by Vachon (1987) found that 48% of the stressors came from the work environment and 29% from factors to do with occupational role. Only 17% came from patient and family contact and 7% from factors relating to the disease. A survey of Macmillan Nurses by Lunt and Yardley (1988) found that 52% expected contacts with other professionals would be stressful, although rather fewer turned out to be so for their sample in practice. From a psychodynamic perspective this might be viewed as an example of displacement. It might be more acceptable to blame external, organizational factors for distress rather than the difficulty of confronting daily the emotional pain, physical distress and pressure to get it right now for those who are dying. Others may bear the responsibility for a failure to live up to high ideals of service, it is not personal. It may also be easier to put into words practical difficulties than more nebulous and philosophical issues. In a survey of the problems perceived by nurses caring for dying people in community, hospice and acute care settings, Copp and Dunn speculated that nurses are more sensitized to perceiving problems of pain for patients and feel more confident in dealing with them. The less tangible spiritual problems were more challenging because there were no protocols for dealing with them and were seldom described by the nurses in their study (Copp and Dunn, 1993).

Environmental stress for staff in specialist settings has been identified as arising from team communication difficulties and conflicts, some of which related to the idealistic aspirations of team members which cannot be realized in practice. In addition there may be tensions between specialist teams and other teams who fail to recognize their expertise and delay referring patients. Vachon (1988) highlighted role ambiguity as one of these environmental stressors. While the role blurring and role overlap which contributes to holistic care can be freeing and stimulating, it can also be experienced as challenging or threatening. She quotes a social worker who said 'things would be a lot better round here if only the physicians would stop talking to the families and leave that to the social worker'. A sad comment which says more about the social worker's needs than about the families' needs. Specialist nurses in palliative care, particularly those working in the community, may develop an expertise in the management of medication and their comparative independence of operation can make this seem a threat to doctors. Some professionals may feel they are giving up more than they are gaining. There is, of course, a positive reason for maintaining watchfulness about what is happening at the boundaries of professional roles. It is important that unsafe practice does not occur. However much a psychologist thinks she understands about nutrition after hearing discussions in ward rounds over many years, it is important to resist the temptation to give advice that comes much better from a nurse who builds it on a depth of training and experience. Similarly a community nurse may develop confidence in talking to children whose parent is dying, but still needs the expertise and knowledge of the social worker to advise on arrangements for future care of the children.

That lower proportion of stresses for specialists in palliative care that are said to be generated from contact with patients and carers arises mainly from those who deal with the illness differently from others, either by extreme anger, denial or withdrawal, or who develop psychiatric symptoms (Vachon, 1995). These difficulties have been discussed in Chapter 4. Studies of those working in more general settings have shown oncology nurses to have a higher rate of burnout and to perceive less support at work than hospice nurses (Bram and Katz, 1989), and that death anxiety is higher among medical and surgical nurses experiencing severe job stress than for hospice nurses (Bene and Foxall, 1991). Dunne and Jenkins (1991) compared stresses and coping strategies for community Macmillan Nurses, hospice nurses, hospital and district nurses, midwives and health visitors working with dying people. They found that 'working exclusively with dying patients is not necessarily more stressful than working with the dying as part of a broader nursing role' and that hospice nurses perceived the least work stress compared with the other groups. The stress for Macmillan Nurses arose as much from inadequate resources and relationships with other professionals, especially GPs, as from patient care.

Vachon (1995) has a plausible explanation for this unexpected finding that in general stress is less in specialist settings than in other settings where dying people are also cared for. She suggests that 'from the earliest days in the hospice movement staff support programmes and team development were seen as integral to effective palliative care'. Paying attention to putting these preventive measures in place has worked. Those that she particularly identifies from research in the field are: developing a team philosophy; team building; a support system at work; developing personal coping strategies. Issues in practice will look in more detail at ways of developing the first three. Personal coping strategies will be considered in the final chapter. However, since many of them relate to working in teams, some discussion of teams and teamwork in palliative care must come first.

7.1.2 Teamwork in palliative care – is it effective?

Teamwork is universally reckoned to be 'a good thing' in health and social care. In palliative care the need to work together springs from the principle of the holistic approach to care and the understanding of total pain described in Chapter 1. No one worker can have all the skills and knowledge necessary. So even if a specialist palliative care service in a hospital or the community starts with just one professional group – most often nurses – they are usually quickly joined by others with a different contribution to make. Is there any evidence that this improves the outcome for the dying person and the carers? Jones' study of 207 people who died at home and their carers provides some confirmation of this (Jones, 1993). Carers were visited two to four months after the death and interviewed by a research nurse. The majority of them had had contact with more than one professional. Teams included any combination of GP, district nurse, specialist palliative care nurse, social worker or other health care professionals. Jones examined how adequately they had been informed about the illness, about local practical support available, and about financial benefits and allowances. He looked at whether they received the domestic help and tuition on simple nursing tasks that they wanted, and how good the symptom control was for pain, constipation, nausea and insomnia. Those visited by the full team including a social worker were much better informed about local support and finance available, and had the lowest unmet need for domestic help. The best symptom relief was achieved when the GP, district nurse and specialist nurse were involved. Seventy four per cent of carers had to carry out simple nursing tasks and the majority had no previous experience to draw on, yet less than half overall received any advice or training in this. The teams that were best at giving this were those already identified. Jones observes that this study did not enquire whether the professionals involved saw themselves as working collaboratively in a team, but nonetheless it does clearly demonstrate that outcomes are improved if a range of skills and knowledge can be brought to bear on the multifaceted problems of dying people and their families. There is less evidence about teams in hospitals, but Knaus and colleagues (1986) looked at the outcomes for patients treated by intensive care teams in 13 hospitals and found that those units that had a high degree of co-ordination had higher survival rates.

7.1.3 Team membership

One of the first questions to be answered is who are to be the members of the team. Jones (1992) and Ajeman (1993), one in the context of primary care, the other in the context of palliative care, plead for teams to be built round tasks rather than structure. So the professional hospice team working on the rehabilitation of someone who has recently become hemiplegic is likely to include as central the physiotherapist and the occupational therapist and the primary nurse. Once discharge becomes a possibility the team must broaden to include the GP, community nurse and social worker. Yet there is likely to be a group of professionals who work together on the problems of the majority of users of any particular service, and who see themselves as having a contribution to make to the overall functioning of the service and not solely a responsibility for their own role.

What about the volunteers and the volunteer organizer? To some extent this will depend on the view in that society on volunteering and the nature of the organization. In the USA volunteers may play a central role in the delivery of health care, in Sweden they are seldom found. In one publicly funded UK hospice the volunteer organizer asked to attend the multi-professional ward-round so that she could have a clearer idea of the needs of patients with whom she would be involving volunteers. This was hotly debated and her continued exclusion seemed to have a symbolic power in representing the value set on volunteers in that setting as handmaidens to the professional team. In the neighbouring independent hospice the volunteer organizer was a member of the management team. Professionals may resent the freedom of the volunteer to pick and choose when they offer their contribution. There may be real anxiety about the substitution of volunteers for tasks previously done by professionals (Relf and Couldrick, 1988). Volunteers may enjoy a close working relationship with professionals in the early days of a service which disappears as the service expands (Field and Johnson, 1993).

Each member of the professional team may have particular issues in relation to their role as team member in addition to the issues around their special skills and knowledge. Those members who are attached to the palliative care team part-time and to another team for the rest of their working week have a difficult balancing act. Each team finds it hard to understand why their need does not have priority. The dynamic nature of palliative care, where the opportunity may be there today but not tomorrow to arrange that final outing or family meeting, adds to the pressure to be available. It is the part-timer who has to manage this and keep the boundaries.

Styles (1994), writing about primary health care teams, highlighted the problems of those supporting members of the team who are less in the public eye, but vital to the functioning of the team. He drew on research on British string quartets to look at the issue of the problems of 'the second violin'. The quartets recognized the need to make decisions democratically, yet there was also a need for leadership. In the quartets those who played second violin were the members who felt most used by the team and who were most likely to leave. The most successful quartets had agreed on the need for a leader, the first violin, but they understood the importance of the subsidiary role and were more complimentary and encouraging to the second violin than the less successful groups. Styles comments 'An important ingredient of success was for individual members to be able to listen to each other and respond to what they heard, and in this way to harmonise their efforts. These skills were different from successful soloists, and indeed could be said to surpass them'.

Roisin, Laval and Lelut (1994) suggest 'It is not a matter of eliminating the difference that must exist within a team, nor of putting oneself in another's place: it is a matter of taking one's own place'. Team members who are confident in what they have to offer and clear about their own role will work more easily and flexibly with the overlap and blurring that a holistic approach demands. The implication of this is that those who have had time to mature in their profession may most easily work in a multiprofessional team.

7.1.4 Are the dying person and their carers members of the team?

Randall and Downie (1996) add another ingredient when they describe the team as 'a changing and flexible group of professionals together with the patient, and often the relatives if they are involved in care or if the patient is incompetent'. They echo early pioneers in the field (Lamerton, 1973). The principle of autonomy certainly should make the patient central to the process and the principle of making those who matter to the patient part of the unit of care joins the carers into the team. However, how successfully do those working in palliative care maintain these principles? The study by Rathbone and colleagues cited in Chapter 4 (Rathbone, Horsley and Goacher, 1994), which found that doctors and nurses missed many of the psychosocial concerns of in-patients in a hospice, shows the importance of including the dying person. It also represents an praiseworthy attempt to put the principles into practice by introducing an assessment for patients to complete on a regular basis. An early comparative study of hospice and showed that doctors in hospices in tne study identified and achieved a wider range of goals for their patients than doctors in the hospital setting. This may provide some indication that dying people and their carers were included.

An interesting study by James (1988) explores the creative tensions between the concepts of 'team' and 'family' as they were used by nurses in an in-patient palliative care unit in the UK to improve their care of dying people. The objective of offering the style of care that would be given by families is frequently found in leaflets of independent hospices (Froggatt, 1995). In James' study nurses used the terms loosely. Either term might sometimes include the patients and their carers. At other times it would be used to describe the staff. The nurses emphasized the team's responsibility for any success and recognized the importance of working to maintain the team. There was some deliberate setting aside of the hierarchical approach which all had experienced in hospital settings, e.g. by asking long-serving auxiliary nurses to induct new trained staff. However, this was only partial, as work was still most frequently allocated by seniority and level of training, and nurses would sometimes call on these old structures as a way of limiting demands on them in time of stress.

The term 'family' was a way of indicating that the ethos of the unit was warm and protective with a different and closer commitment between its members from that found in other health-care settings. It was an ethos which allowed for more open expression of emotion and greater familiarity between members, though there were varying ideas about where to draw the line in the relationship with patients. It enabled the nurse to reflect what standard of care she would want to offer one of her own family and act on it here. However, James points out the difficulties of marrying the potential unlimited remit of the care families offer each other with the accountability and set professional roles of the staff. Family care is domestic, private and on a small scale, deriving from relationships usually built up over some time. Staff must spread their caring over large numbers, even with the advent of the primary nurse, and over a short time. If routinization and bureaucratization are indeed increasing in palliative care (James and Field, 1992), then this is an area needing especial vigilance. More work is needed to explore the implications of the inclusion of dying person and carer in the team in today's systems of health and social care.

7.1.5 Issues for teams

Teams have to decide how to balance co-ordination and good communication with action. Ajeman (1993) suggests that there is a series of questions that should be asked to determine how decisions are made, to avoid both the inefficiency of including everyone in the team all the time and the failures if key information is not available.

- Who has the information necessary to make the decision?
- Who needs to be consulted before the decision is made?
- Who needs to be informed of the decision after it is made?

Regular well-organized team meetings can help to establish both general principles for decision making which all agree on and the trust in each other which can sustain the team through an emergency when there is too little time for widespread consultation. In community teams only one member may be visiting the home, but they need to carry with them a sense of taking the resources of the whole team with them, so that they remain alert to the possibility of involving other members, either in person or as a consultant to the work they are doing on their own.

There can be a danger for a group of people who work together most of the time becoming too inward looking in their attempt to develop cohesion. Randall and Downie (1996) discuss the moral issues raised by the intellectually 'cosy' or introverted team where the team becomes more important than the dying person. It may exclude those who become too challenging or fail to draw in those elsewhere in the community or institution whose skills are needed in a particular situation. Despite the increased prevalence of psychiatric disorders in those with terminal cancer compared with those with earlier stages of the disease (Breitbart and Passik, 1993) and the stress that working with psychiatrically ill patients brings for staff, relatively few psychiatrists have a regular link with specialist palliative care services. Ways of maintaining openness can be a good staff development programme and each team member keeping close links with their own professional organization.

In every team leadership is a central issue. West (1990) makes a distinction between the manager of the team who ensures day-to-day continuity and the leader of the team who may be different depending on the particular problem and decision required. These two roles must be well co-ordinated. Randall and Downie (1996) consider whether the collective responsibility that palliative care principles imply is real. They acknowledge that what is most frequently found is the situation where all members of the team contribute in varying degrees to a discussion on managing the problems of the dying person and their carers but the final accountability rests with the one professional responsible for that area of care. They plead, however for an emerging multiprofessional responsibility where 'a conscientious compromise is reached which all the professionals feel they can support ideologically and practically'. How to handle the conflicts that occur when such a compromise cannot be reached will be considered in the Issues in practice section.

7.1.6 Advocacy

How does the idea of a professional acting as advocate for the patient square with the multiprofessional responsibility around a conscientious compromise, put forward as the ideal by Randall and Downie? Nurses and social workers have particularly identified themselves as advocates for patients – the nurse often in relation to the powerful doctor, the social worker in relation to powerful institutions like the Department of Social Security. Webber suggests that three factors have contributed to the increased emphasis on the nurse as advocate for the patient – the more equal position of women in society in general, greater recruitment of men into nursing and individualized patient care (Webber, 1987). However, Penn is cautious about how realistic it is for a nurse to act in this way for those who are dying (Penn, 1994). Communication barriers may exist between nurses and palliative care patients (Wilkinson, 1991) and there is no guarantee that the patient will perceive the nurse as any less threatening than the doctor.

Certainly Randall and Downie set out the pitfalls of one member of the team identifying themselves or being identified as the patient's advocate while others are not. What if the patient seeks an objective which the advocate feels might be harmful? What say do patients have in who shall be their advocate? In the fields of mental health, learning disability and the care of older people citizen advocacy schemes are developing which use trained lay people to act as advocates. If this happens in palliative care will it signal that the professionals in the field have been thoroughly routinized and bureaucratized? Or will it be a recognition that the role of advocate and multiprofessional team member can sit uncomfortably together? It is one of the few disadvantages of working in teams that they have the potential to reduce choice for the dying person and their carer precisely through the compromise agreed on by the team as the best way of proceeding (Lonsdale *et al.*, 1980).

7.2 ISSUES IN PRACTICE

7.2.1 Team building

Iles and Auluck (1990) recommend that teams attend, in order of priority, to developing common goals, clarifying roles and procedures, and improving team relationships. Working to a common purpose may be assisted by a common language (Roisin, Laval and Lelut, 1994). However, this does not necessarily mean giving up cherished and significant words, but does mean understanding and respecting why the term for the same individual may be 'patient' for the doctor, 'client' for the psychologist and 'service user' for the social worker. Developing common purpose can take place at a number of levels. A new team must consciously work at developing a philosophy of care and a set of specific goals. This may begin the process of developing a common language. Once these are established they require regular reviews which take into account both changes in the context of the team's work, like the introduction of health care purchasing, or changes in team personnel. Such reviews must take place at sessions separate from those meetings planning individual patient care so that the focus is clear. Doing a SWOT analysis – listing the team's Strengths, Weaknesses, Opportunities and Threats – can be a useful tool here. Teams must have a clear system for integrating new members. Teams are dynamic, and as a new member joins and works their way into the team their contribution will alter an emphasis or add a goal. The recruitment of a nurse in an in-patient hospice who had trained in children's nursing brought about a much clearer recognition of the needs of patients' children and grandchildren in the setting, and fostered a much improved co-operation with the social worker in the team over their care. Part of the regular review must consider the life-cycle of the team. Ways of working and styles of leadership that suit a well-established team of mature professionals may need to be revised if there is a sudden influx of new members who are at an early stage of their career.

However, common purpose and common language also emerge from actually working together and attempting to make real the philosophy and goals of the team in relation to this dying person and their carers. So the team leader or manager will particularly need to have their eye on the philosophy and goals in ward or clinical team meetings to discuss patient care, and encourage the team to test proposed actions against them. Since what is being communicated is not simply information about the individual's work but also their personal response to their involvement with this particular client or patient and to death and dying, Jackson (1990) points out that it is important that those present should feel safe to express this. Regular weekly meetings at a set time and of a defined length will contribute to this, but valuing team members and maintaining self-esteem through praise and feedback is crucial. Permission to acknowledge difficulties is essential. The doctor needs to be able to say that he finds it very hard to listen to Mrs Jones' complaints about her hard-working GP; the nurse needs to be able to confess that meeting an alcoholic carer was particularly challenging. She comments 'A good team is able to accept the weaknesses as well as the strengths of each member, recognizing its own frailties and learning from others. How vital for a team of "experts" to acknowledge their humanity'. Developing good procedures should not be neglected. A primary health care team focusing on improving their care for dying people found that the simple expedient of instituting a book in which the social worker could leave messages for the rest of the team greatly improved the co-ordination of care.

If role ambiguity is a potential problem in specialist palliative care as we saw in Setting the scene, then working on clarifying roles is time well spent. Iles and Auluck (1990) give examples of approaches to doing this. One is where a professional initiates an analysis of their role, its rationale and duties, and this is added to or altered until both the person who has the role and the rest of the group agree that the description fits the role. Other roles in the team are then analyzed in turn. Another approach is for each team member to draw up three lists, the first of the things they like and value about the others in the group, the second of what they would like other members of the group to change about the way they work, and a third predicting what items other members of the group might be putting in their lists about them and their role. This last list is an attempt to bring out into the open some of the fears and fantasies that we all have what others think of us, and which may be inaccurate but nonetheless a powerful influence on our response to them. Another aspect of clarifying roles may be to recognize the different roles played by different members of the team in carrying out the team's business. Belbin's view is that 'imperfect people make perfect teams' and that there are eight team roles that together contribute to a team functioning well (Belbin, 1981). By using an exercise like the Belbin Team Roles exercise individuals can identify whether their main contribution is, for example, as the person who generates new ideas, the person who ensures that projects are completed or the person who sees that the team has the right information. Any exercises looking at clarifying roles are best carried out with a facilitator who is trusted by the team, but not a member of it, and who brings an independent view which may help the group to move forward rather than remain stuck in unhelpful stereotyping.

7.2.2 Joint education

One potential contributor to building the team is learning together with other professionals. This may be through the team having study days together or through other education and training events which have multi-professional participation. Increasingly there are attempts to develop joint education at qualifying level and Coles (1996) thinks that specialist palliative care, with its often well-developed team working and its theory base drawn from practice, could make a significant contribution here. One report identifies a rationale for multiprofessional education – 'by sharing skills, experiences and attitudes the undergraduate students or professionals in continuing education get an insight in [sic] similarities and dissimilarities between the different health professions. An increased respect and mutual understanding of each other is thus facilitated' (Council of Europe, 1995). Given that such improvements in respect and understanding do not happen just through sitting a mixed group of professionals in a room together, what conditions will help this to take place?

First, value what all students, at whatever level, bring. Coles observes 'The educational process, rather than being technical training, is more concerned with development, and acknowledges that the learners bring a considerable amount of knowledge and experience with them, which can usefully form the basis of their education. Whilst teachers may know a lot, they recognize that little can be gained merely by transmitting knowledge, but rather enable learners to learn through a co-operative and collaborative dialogue' (Coles, 1996). Second, teachers from different health and social care professions who enjoy teaching together can model good collaborative working and show that it is possible to open up the discussion of difficult areas. Third, working on education projects together can develop trust and mutual respect (Council of Europe, 1995). As part of a joint training day on palliative care, nursing and medical students were required to interview the carer of someone who was dying together. This had to be done sensitively to avoid distress to the carer. The facilitators felt that sharing the responsibility for this was freeing and allowed a great deal of learning to take place. The evaluations of the day were very positive. Nash and Hoy (1993) found that workshops on terminal care in the community for pairs of GPs and District Nurses from the same practice, using an action learning approach with case studies, small group discussion and project work, resulted in increased co-operation and confidence in the delivery of palliative care. Fourth, teachers must recognize the personal resonance that the issues being discussed in palliative care education may have for participants and ensure that they feel safe either in sharing these or in keeping silent. There may be important parallels to be drawn between the experience of learners in taking the risk of exposing themselves to learning perhaps with an unfamiliar group and the experience of the dying person making contact with a palliative care service (Sheldon and Smith, 1996).

7.2.3 Support systems

In the early days of palliative care staff support groups were sometimes seen as the only answer to meeting support needs. Now it is increasingly recognized that a number of different factors contribute to a climate which helps staff to continue to stand alongside despairing and distressed people. Good recruitment and induction policies, clear job descriptions, managers who are seen to be working to secure adequate resources for the service, all demonstrate that the organization values its staff. Opportunities for education and training provide days away from confronting the sadness of dying people and their carers directly, and give new stimulation and a breathing space for reflection and review. To be most useful these should form part of a planned programme of development to improve practice, based on regular appraisal with a manager or team leader, not just be a flight from painful reality. Vachon's review (1995) showed that many research studies identify 'talking things over with a colleague' as one of the most widely used and effective coping mechanisms, often more valuable than seeking support from family or friends. Dunne and Jenkins (1991) found that Macmillan Nurses relied heavily on informal support from colleagues in dealing with work stress. Monroe (1993b) reminds us of the importance of endings, and of managing and marking endings in this work. Different settings will approach this differently. For some it may be common to attend funerals of former patients in work time, for others this is a luxury that shortage of staff and the demands of those still living does not allow. Yet for every professional there is every now and again a funeral of someone to whom they have become close that must be attended if they are to be able to continue their commitment to palliative care. Unless organizations recognize this they risk losing experienced staff. An audit of care which makes an assessment of how the care has gone for each person who dies, memorial services and the existence of good bereavement after-care are other ways of respecting endings.

7.2.4 Staff support groups

Support groups can make a valuable contribution to supporting staff but there are certain principles to follow and issues to consider to ensure this happens. Alexander has set these out succinctly (Alexander, 1993).

Clear aims

These are professional groups which should be work-related and purpose driven. They may be aimed at giving an opportunity for expressing feelings and ideas in a safe setting, at producing constructive feedback from the group on work issues for individual group members, or at offering guidance on ways of coping with stress at work. Groups are most effective when members decide the emphasis they wish this group to have and the way it should work within these parameters.

Membership

Groups of one profession only may feel safe but may suffer from too narrow a focus and a tendency to scapegoat other groups. For groups with too wide a range of professionals and non-professionals it may be difficult to find common ground. The mix in the group and the advantages and disadvantages of different mixes should be carefully considered before the start, and attention should be paid to ensuring that those not included do not feel excluded or unprivileged. If numbers are too great some members may feel too intimidated to contribute, if too small some may feel too exposed. Alexander (1993) recommends between eight and 12 members as a workable number. Membership should not be imposed. Senior staff in a specialist palliative care setting identified a need for a staff support group and leaned heavily on staff to attend, but did not attend themselves. This was interpreted by group members as the senior staff thinking 'We senior staff are tough and able to take it, but you junior lot are weak and can't cope'. This caused considerable resentment which caused the group to abort and continued to sour relationships.

Group life-cycle

It is important to consider before the start of the group how long it is intended to run for and whether during that period it should be open to new members joining or whether membership should be closed after the first session. Closed groups more easily develop a stable identity and agreed way of working, but may be unrealistic in settings where there are large numbers of staff and some degree of turnover. Vachon's review of research (1995) suggests that time-limited groups are most helpful. So even if a support group is intended to be a regular part of the staff support system it may be appropriate to have a break, say over the summer holiday period, so that the group has an opportunity to take on a new form or different membership more easily.

Leadership

There is a need for the boundaries of the group's functioning to be well-managed. Keeping to agreed times, ensuring a proper place to meet, keeping the group focused are all tasks that to some extent must be shared by all group members, but a leader can take particular responsibility for them. Alexander (1993) suggests that a leader must be flexible, command respect, have professional standing and preferably be from outside the group so that they can take a more detached view. The objective is to help the group to work, neither to dominate nor to be passive. For this reason the leader should not feel obliged to solve all the problems presented by the group members or feel solely responsible for maintaining the group. Groups may often seek to give this responsibility to the leader, but it should be handed firmly back to them. The convenor of a support group for palliative care nurses felt under pressure to decide whether it should continue as it was or invite speakers to meetings. The group was polarized on this issue. After discussion with a groupwork consultant she handed the decision back to group members. Once they saw that she would not make the decision they were perfectly well able to come to a compromise that was satisfactory to them all.

Group rules

These must be discussed and agreed at the start of the group and the leader, if there is one, or some other member, must take responsibility for ensuring that those who join later know what they are. Group rules contribute to the sense of safety which group members must have if discussion is to have any depth. A fundamental rule is to keep confidential to group members material that is discussed within the group. Ann, a nurse in a support group of oncology nurses told the others that a colleague not in the group had commented to her that she had heard that Julie, another group member, had become upset at the previous session. Although the comment was reported as showing concern and a wish to help Julie, there was anger and consternation in the group. They now felt exposed, the more so as it was not possible to establish with certainly who was responsible for the breach of confidentiality. Only two members turned up for the subsequent session. Other rules regarding time keeping, only one person speaking at a time, respect for all contributions, set the tone. The group leader may need to help some quieter or less confident members to speak on occasion, but they should not be pressurised to speak. Listeners are as much needed in a group as talkers. However, if they never speak they may need to be helped to see that other group members may wonder what they are thinking, and may interpret their silence as threatening or hostile.

7.2.5 Handling conflict in teams

Conflict in teams can be creative, producing new solutions to problems, or it can be destructive, creating bitterness and resentment. 'Interdisciplinary working uncovers blind spots within the team that could become a source of injury and psychological anguish' (Roisin, Laval and Lelut, 1994). However, one report on the effect of the hospice experience on the church's ministry of healing commented 'if there is no conflict, there is almost certainly no true teamwork [but merely] parallel professional practice' (Twycross, R. [ed.], *Mud and Stars*, quoted in Copp and Dunn, 1993). So the trick is not 'how to avoid conflict but to manage it so that it enriches the programme' (Ajeman, 1993). Conflict may emerge from underlying issues such as the role ambiguity and overlap in palliative care discussed earlier, different priorities for different team members especially where resources are scarce, barriers arising from the separate organizational structures of health and social care in the UK, the status of different team members and the leadership style of the team leader. Personality differences play their part. Common flash points for conflict in palliative care teams are: decisions about discharge from specialist in-patient units – the nurses doubtful about the possibility of this patient managing nights alone at home, the doctor trying to balance the competing needs of patients already in beds and those in the community unknown to the in-patient team but desperately needing help; disagreements about the appropriate levels of pain control or sedation – the latter particularly for anxious patients near death; how to balance the interests of the patient who longs to go home or to stay at home and those of a carer who no longer wishes to care.

Randall and Downie remind us that one principle must underpin the approach to resolving conflict. 'Respect for the autonomy of others demands that we recognize that they may have moral values which differ from our own, and therefore we respect their right to reach different conclusions in clinical decisions' (Randall and Downie, 1996). An appre-ciation of the underlying issues detailed above which may be contributing to the conflict helps in understanding why, for example, a disagreement between the doctor and the social worker about discharge may be so passionately felt. The doctor may feel impotent now the Department of Social Services controls the budget for nursing home and community care in the UK which may limit the clinical options, the social worker may resent the doctor's status and higher income.

The principle of patient autonomy can help to unlock some conflicts. Miss Brown, whose cancer had badly affected her ability to get up from a chair, who could not stand or walk even short distances without a supporting frame, wanted to return to live alone in her neglected tumble-down house with uneven floors and no downstairs lavatory. She scorned the occupational therapist's aids and preferred to devise her own mech-anism for pulling herself out of a chair with an old piece of rope. She insisted that in time she would walk independently again and drive her car. The occupational therapy aide who had accompanied her on a home visit was convinced she would be in danger at home. The social worker helped the team to focus on Miss Brown's right to take risks and to die alone at home as a result of an accident, provided that team members had expressed their anxieties to her. She did return home for some months with some paid home care support which she would allow only a strictly limited remit and at one time managed to walk independently round the ground floor. She asked to return to the hospice about a week before her death, only acknowledging that she needed a short break. She seemed to feel able to come in again because her rights had previously been respected.

If teams have spent time on developing and maintaining a team philos-ophy, and on team building destructive conflicts are less likely to arise. It is worth examining some of the common 'flashpoint' issues at team study days where they can be discussed around case examples but not in the context of a particular case where passions are already aroused and battle lines drawn up. West recommends that if ethical or personality clashes do still arise at moments of crisis when time and staff are in short supply, and work is pouring in, it is better for the team leader to call a full team meeting to discuss the issue and resolve it rather than skate over it and let it fester until a less hectic moment (West, 1993).

Ajeman (1993) has useful guidelines for resolving conflict with a colleague or between two parties. For two colleagues she recommends:

- Allowing emotions to cool a little.
- Choosing a private spot to put over what you think has happened and why it was difficult for you but doing so in a way which respects the self-respect and dignity of the other person.
- Describing the change you would like to see, what positive effects you think it would have.
- Listening to other possible solutions advanced by your colleague.
- Agreeing to settle on one solution and review it after an agreed time.

If the conflict is between two groups a third party respected by both may help to clarify what the issues are, develop ways of working on those issues which generate as many solutions as possible, identify goals and if the solution lies at levels in the organization beyond the two groups in conflict. Again a key principle is to do all this in a way that preserves individual's self-esteem and dignity and acknowledges, without patronizing, the personal cost of any compromise.

7.3 CONCLUSION

As we have seen, working in teams can create stress but also buffer against it. This is true of so many support mechanisms. Joining in social events is often advocated as a way of team building and reducing stress, but for some this may be experienced as very stressful as they wonder what to wear, how to talk to the doctor with whom conversation was so easy in the defined context of work but much more stilted in the restaurant or theatre. Perhaps the best approach to working together is to try to maintain your faith in yourself as a competent professional by ensuring that your contribution is as good as you can make it, but to retain a humility which recognizes no one profession or professional has a monopoly on excellence. Above all, welcome and enjoy the stimulation which working with other professionals in palliative care with different perspectives can bring.

<table>
<tr><td>8</td><td># Living with dying</td></tr>
</table>

This book is about how professionals may most helpfully stand alongside people who are dealing with transition and change, whether that is their own death or the death of another who is intimately interwoven with their life. There are so many uncertainties for all the participants to face. Reimer and her colleagues (Reimer, Davis and Martens, 1991) identified the time of transition when families first realize that death is coming close as 'the neutral zone', a time of emptiness when the old familiar reality was gone and nothing looked solid any more. They comment 'The central struggle of the neutral zone had to do with the paradox of living and dying at the same time'. So how to live with dying is a question for the dying person, their carers and the professional teams. How long will this time of transition last? Within the global overall change what are the smaller changes that people are likely to encounter and may begin to prepare for – physical, psychological, relational? Can we make sense of what is happening, whether we are the person who is dying, the person who is bereaved or the professional in touch with either? Does it matter if we can or cannot make sense of it? How can we be sure that the services we are offering are appropriate and of a high enough standard?

In this chapter we return to the principles of palliative care and the key concepts outlined in Chapter 1, and consider how they may be expressed in ways beyond the conventional approaches to delivering health and social care. A holistic approach gives scope for including the role of the arts and of complementary therapies both for the dying person and their carers, and for the professional. Both may contribute to quality of life, and may enable explorations of what autonomy can be when physical and intellectual powers may be failing, may enable too the painful search for meaning for any of the players in the story. Finally we look at the issue of quality in palliative care. We begin by considering the personal toll for the professional working alongside dying people and their carers, continuing the theme of the previous chapter but concentrating on the individual rather than on the interactions with others.

8.1 PREVENTING BURNOUT AND BATTLE FATIGUE

Vachon (1995) has demonstrated that the popular preconception that working with dying people must necessarily be more stressful than other areas of health care is incorrect. Burnout, 'the progressive loss of idealism, energy and purpose experienced by people in the helping professions as a result of the conditions of their work' (Edelwich and Brodsky, 1980, cited in Vachon, 1995), has been found to be less common in hospice staff when they have been compared with mental health workers or oncology nurses. As we have seen Vachon's explanation is that specialist settings have paid attention to staff support. Despite this individuals may from time to time feel helpless and useless at their failure to ensure 'a good death' for particular patients, and depressed about the multiple losses that they experience. For those working in generalist settings it may be even more testing. Jane Martin records how when a busy new junior doctor she had to deal with the death of her father in another hospital similar to the one she worked in, and how difficult it seemed to be for the hospital who employed her to allow her to be vulnerable and for her to remain in touch with her human feelings. 'In re-donning the white coat, it seemed, I had covered up my claim to be a human being with the capacity to be hurt and the right to crawl away and lick my wounds' (Martin, 1989). Vachon identifies an important point before burnout occurs when the result of cumulative exposure to the suffering and deaths of large numbers of patients and grieving carers produces 'battle fatigue' (Vachon, 1988). Continuing the analogy, she suggests that, though a brief break from the trenches of specialist palliative care may be necessary, there can then be time for consideration of how the stresses can be reduced so that there can be a return to the fray. In the last chapter we considered what teams can do to sustain themselves and their members. What are the most effective personal strategies that individual professionals can employ ?

When Davies and Oberle (1990) analysed the elements of the supportive role of the nurse in palliative care, they found that for the home care nurses they studied in the western USA the core dimension round which all the others were integrated was that of preserving their own integrity. Without working on this they could not carry out other aspects of the role more directly concerned with patients. They did this by maintaining self-awareness and a critical approach to their own practice, by using techniques to maintain an appropriate distance such as humour and by sharing frustrations with colleagues. In a study of the role of the specialist social worker in palliative care in the UK using a similar methodology (Sheldon, unpublished), recognizing that there are limits, whether those are the limits of life itself, of individual personalities or of resources, and working creatively within limits was the dimension that enabled the social worker to knit together the other parts of the role. Mesler (1994–95) too found that hospice staff were clear that they must set limits to their working day and to their emotional involvement to continue to work in the setting. So one strategy is that of taking your own responsibility for monitoring and maintaining the balance between over-involvement and remoteness. The use of supervision or consultation to assist in this process is well-established in social work, and nurses will have the benefit of this too, once clinical supervision takes hold in the UK. It is particularly important for those working as single representatives of their profession in a team, where it is crucial to maintain a sense of the particular contribution that your profession can make, or for those specialists in palliative care working alone in a hospital or in the community, as happens sometimes in the early days of a specialist service.

8.2 THE ROLE OF THE ARTS

Ways of exploring the deeper meaning of being in this time of transition can go beyond the exchange of words in counselling sessions or the staff support group. The Art in Hospitals programme in the UK, which has transformed many long corridors and gloomy waiting rooms with murals and mobiles, is a recognition of the way the environment contributes to patient morale and thus to recovery. Bertman (1991) claims a role for the arts in the arena of palliative care. She suggests that the arts can:

- Increase understanding of psychosocial and existential issues related to death, dying and grief and stimulate more sensitive observations of the human condition.
- Provide an arena for the generation of creative options and problem solving possibilities for patients, family members, and health care professionals.
- Assist education
- Encourage alliances between the medical community, other human sciences and the arts.

In one example, through developing a programme of mainly visual images of death and encouraging students to create their own images, she enabled medical students to approach their first experience of dissection not just as a mechanical and distant experience but in a way that integrated their humanity with the need to develop technical skill and knowledge. One student wrote afterwards:

> Dissection isn't:
> cadavers coming to life
> desecrating the dead
> hurting the person
> for fun

appalling
unethical
sadistic
pleasant
bad for you
casual

Dissection is:
part of learning medicine
interesting
reflective
accepting a gift
group experience
a rite of passage
probably smelly
something hard

From Bertman, S. (1991) *Facing Death: Images, Insights and Interventions*, p. 131, Taylor and Francis, Washington, DC. Reproduced with permission. All rights reserved.

The thoughtful seriousness and balance of this 'verbal collage', as Bertman calls it, captures the essence of the way that using the arts in education can develop understanding for those who are, or will be, working close to death.

Of course, many professionals make use of the arts, particularly music and literature, not just in the classroom but in their personal lives, maybe as a route to relaxation or to taking off the burdens of the day, maybe as a comfort or way of transcending the pain and despair about them. Sometimes it is only through the arts that the complexity of human emotion and relationships which we work with can be satisfactorily encapsulated. The poem *The Widow's Complaint* conveys the rage and passionate ambivalence of love and hate which are common feelings in bereavement but seldom so succinctly expressed.

The Widow's Complaint

You left as you so often left before
Sneaking out on tiptoe
No slam of door,
Off to drink with enemies of mine,
And of yours –
If you could only see it –
Drunkards and bores
Whose grossest flatteries
You swilled down with the booze

That you never had the gumption to refuse.
You won't come back this time.
No need to prepare a welcome for you – clamped silence
And belligerent stare –
No need for morning nostrums or to hide
The whiskey and the car keys,
Tighten lips and thighs
Against your pleas.

No need for those old stratagems any more.
But you might have let me know what was in store;
Your last low trick
To leave me with no clue that you had gone for good,
My last chance lost
To tell you what I've so long wanted to,
How much I hate you and I always have,
You pig, you bastard,
Stinking rat –
O love, my love, how can I forgive you that?

Reproduced with permission from Vernon Scannell, *Collected Poems 1950–1993*. Published by Robson Books.

It is, however, in initiatives which enable people who are dying or bereaved to develop their experience and use of the arts, perhaps for the first time, that provide perhaps the most fruitful examples in this area – generating the creative options and problem-solving possibilities of which Bertman speaks. Frampton (1993) suggests that a palliative care arts programme can improve feelings of personal worth and purpose for the dying person at a time when these are often in short supply, and this may happen particularly through creating something to leave behind. Mayo (1996) thinks that art therapy may be able to start to answer the question 'Why me?' and describes two case studies where a man and a woman, each with very different histories and approaches to life, using this medium find a way to gain access to their unconscious life and achieve a degree of resolution of issues in their lives. Alida Gersie, in her book *Storymaking in Bereavement: Dragons Fight in the Meadow* (1991), describes ways of using stories from many cultures and times as a stimulus to creative work in therapeutic groups for bereaved people. Such activities can range from exploring ideas and feelings through the medium of the arts where they are a resource available to the dying or bereaved person (Frampton, 1993) to art or music therapy being carried out by a trained therapist. It is particularly important for those who are not professionally trained in this field to refrain from attempting to interpret the meaning of what a dying person or carer produces. What it signifies for them is what is important.

From the early days of palliative care there have been centres which have included the arts as an important part of the therapeutic programme. The Royal Victoria Hospital in Montreal employed a music therapist and she reported reduced physical symptoms and use of medication in patients treated, as well as a sense of spiritual comfort (Munro and Mount, 1978). The Royal Marsden Cancer Hospital established an art therapy service as part of its rehabilitation programme (Connell, 1992) and the charity Hospice Arts has funded a number of initiatives in the UK. This charity has also attempted the difficult task of evaluating the value and effectiveness of arts projects in palliative care. One such evaluation did demonstrate that projects are unlikely to be successful unless patients feel involved from the start and can help shape the project (McIllmurray *et al.*, 1992). One intervention in which art therapists have often been involved are the groups for bereaved children described in Chapter 6.

8.3 COMPLEMENTARY THERAPIES

The growth of interest in complementary therapies and their relationship with conventional health care has been a fascinating aspect of western health care in the last part of the 20th century. That relationship has been particularly fraught in cancer care. There was a period of outright hostility when complementary therapies were more often described as 'alternative' with all that implied about being in opposition to conventional medical care. This has been succeeded by a period of much greater co-operation and a recognition that holistic care may require both. Indeed the boundaries between the two are continually shifting. Some therapies once thought of as 'unscientific' like acupuncture now have ' a sound scientific basis and clinical credibility' and the dignity of a section in the *Oxford Textbook of Palliative Medicine* (Thompson and Filshie, 1993). Complementary therapies have been a common feature of palliative care services for people with AIDS in the UK (Small, 1993). Penson (1991) divides the complementary therapies most commonly used in palliative care into two groups: those that require extensive training to practice like homeopathy and acupuncture, and those that can easily be incorporated into nursing care like massage and relaxation. Of course such therapies or other medical practices such as Chinese medicine may still be used by some patients as an alternative rather than as complementary to conventional care.

Studies of the proportion of cancer patients using complementary therapies show wide variation from 16% in a study by Downer and colleagues in the UK (Downer *et al.*, 1994) to 54% reported by Cassileth in the USA (Cassileth *et al.*, 1984). The latter considers the cultural factors which underlie the increased interest in such therapies and suggests that it stems from the movement for patients' rights and consumer choice in health care, a mistrust of organized medicine with its biomedical model and a growing emphasis on fitness and taking personal responsibility for remaining healthy. Clearly the different cultures of the UK and the USA give different weight to different factors. In the UK those who have sought complementary therapies in cancer care have often done so because they wanted to feel more in control and less passively dependent on doctors, and that they were making a contribution to their own cure or care (Brohn, 1987). What those who use them also describe is a feeling of being valued and cared for: 'The whole experience (the massage) made me feel I was worth caring about' (Corner, Cawley and Hildebrand, 1995). This may be because so many of the most common, like massage, aromatherapy, reflexology, use touch. The use of touch by nurses has been shown to increase patients' perceptions that a nurse was interested in their well-being (Weiss, 1988).

How to evaluate the effectiveness of complementary therapies has been a contentious issue and Anthony (1993) sets out some of the difficulties involved – the individually designed treatment for each patient, the recognition of the importance of what the patient brings in the shape of constitution, personality and history, how to isolate the effects of the therapy from other factors. Studies comparing massage and aromatherapy are a nice example of this. Corner and her colleagues (1995) attempted to do this in a rehabilitation centre at a cancer hospital by comparing three groups, a group offered massage alone, a group offered massage with a blend of essential oils and a control group who had neither. While they found that anxiety but not depression, was significantly reduced for those in both massage groups, symptoms improved for all groups over the course of the study. Patients were positive about the interventions and half directly attributed improvements in their physical symptoms to the massage. The authors conclude 'Massage and a number of other therapies are holistic and involve many interacting elements. The effects of massage as a form of touch are indistinguishable from the relationship the patient may establish with the massage therapist, or from the environment in which the massage takes place'. They recommend that further research should try through a combination of methodological approaches to assess the different contributions of the different elements but should also be concerned to maintain a holistic evaluation.

One common consequence of therapies like massage being introduced for patients in palliative care settings is that staff request sessions for themselves. They perceive a benefit for patients, whether or not effectiveness is demonstrated by research. So complementary therapies may form part of the programme of staff support to reduce stress. Mathers (1995) particularly recommends relaxation and breathing techniques for this purpose, to help nurses restore physiological and psychological balance.

8.4 ASSURING QUALITY

In the early days of the development of specialist palliative care it seemed almost to be taken for granted that standards were high and that care was appropriate (McKee, 1993). Higginson (1992) and Ingleton and Faulkner (1994) both identify a certain hostility by professionals to the whole notion of quality assurance and especially to one of its manifestations, audit. There is some confusion about what it is, some anxiety about criticism that may emerge from an assessment of the quality of care, and perhaps a belief that anyway outcomes in palliative care are not susceptible to measurement because of their qualitative and holistic nature. Sometimes a discussion about quality can seem dry and abstract, even simplistic, not connected to the messy and complex business of looking after real human beings. Nevertheless, as specialist palliative care becomes more incorporated into general health and social care and purchasers seek for evidence of effectiveness and quality in the services they purchase, it cannot ignore the general trend towards a focus on quality assurance. Nor can professionals in palliative care assume that because they aspire to high standards they will necessarily achieve them. The gratitude so often expressed by dying people and their carers may be misleading. Just as in any other branch of health and social care their expectations may be very low and they may be fearful of alienating those on whom they depend for care.

Commonly accepted elements of a high quality service are that it should be appropriate, accessible, effective, the most efficient use of the resources devoted to the service and delivered equitably to all who need it (Ingleton and Faulkner, 1994). We have considered some of the issues around equity and access in Chapters 1 and 3 particularly. Ingleton and Faulkner (1994) add continuity and co-ordination of care, and how acceptable care is to those providing it, as other important dimensions in quality in palliative care. This last dimension matters because staff who are constantly striving to improve what they do are likely to do better than those who are complacent. Wilkinson's study of nurse communication showed that those nurses who were most concerned to maintain high standards were those who least used blocking tactics with patients (Wilkinson, 1991). Quality may be fostered by external mechanisms such as the minimum standards laid down by Health Authorities for the registration of independent hospices as private nursing homes, accreditation by the Royal Colleges as a setting that is permitted to train doctors and medical students or an organizational audit by external assessors such as that developed by Cancer Relief Macmillan Fund (1994). These approaches to quality most often consider the structure, that is the resources allocated to the service like staff and beds, and the processes by which the service is delivered like procedures and throughput, rather than the outcomes of the service.

However, one of the most common approaches to ensuring that a quality service is being delivered is through a review of clinical care against agreed standards, which is more likely to look at outcomes, though it may also be interested in the process of care as a proxy for outcomes that are difficult to measure. So an audit of a bereavement service may consider what proportion of bereaved receive a contact by phone or in person within the first month after the death, rather than what the outcome of their bereavement is at one month. This process of audit requires that first a standard is defined which is based on best current practice. Then the aspect of care is monitored against the standard and any deficiencies in practice are put right. This is the ideal. In practice there are a number of hurdles.

First there may not be an agreed standard for, say, spiritual care. This may then require a piece of research to determine what best practice should be. This brings in another issue – that of including the perspectives of the dying person and their carers. We have looked at some of the principles and research around this in Chapters 1 and 5. The authors in the most comprehensive book so far on audit in palliative care (Higginson, 1993b) do not always make clear how this is included. Yet if it is not a basic principle of palliative care is eroded. Dying people have an interest in the audit of even the most apparently objective and scientific aspect of care. How invasive is the procedure which produces the result? How often must they have it? How sensitively was it delivered? Hopkins (1993) reminds us that it is ethically wrong to persist with professional practice that has not been evaluated and this supports the need for audit. However, it is also important that dying people are not subjected to procedures in the name of audit, such as questionnaires or interviews of a type which, if they were being administered as part of a research project, would have been rejected by a Local Research Ethics Committee. Those involved in audit must carefully balance the importance of including the dying person with respecting their vulnerability.

Then too those carrying out audit should not fall into the trap of 'acquiring information because it is easily measured (e.g. respiration rates) even though the data do not determine the outcomes of patient care' (Hopkins, 1993). Audit in palliative care requires both quantitative and qualitative approaches to assess holistic and multi professional care. One tool which has now been widely tested and adapted to different settings is the Support Team Assessment Schedule (STAS) developed by Higginson and colleagues (Higginson, Wade and McCarthy, 1992) originally to assess the work of Community Support Teams. The original version used 17 key indicators of palliative care which were given a rating each week by staff involved in care (a shorter version is now available). They found it difficult to complete items assessing spiritual care and financial matters, but those on symptom control, pain control, communication between professionals, and communication from professionals to patients and family were rarely missed (Higginson, Wade and McCarthy, 1992). A criticism of this tool is that it does not include the assessment of the dying person in relation to the items. When Higginson and McCarthy (1993) examined how closely staff ratings reflected those of patients and carers, they found that staff ratings were most often closer to family members than to the ratings of the patient about the seven items that they looked at in the STAS. Patients rated themselves as less anxious then either of the other two groups and family members saw more problems than others. However, we saw in Chapter 5 that this reflects the reality that each individual will necessarily see the same situation from their own perspective and therefore differently. Provided those who are using it are aware of the possible biases, it does have the advantage that, because it is staff rated, it can be used for patients who are very sick or do not have carers.

A qualitative approach that has become popular is the focus group. Focus groups bring together a group of people who have a common interest or common experience. A skilled group facilitator, using a standardized set of questions and neutral probes, helps them develop a discussion which provides information on the topic of concern. Woodward and King (1993) report on using this method with carers of patients who had recently died at Chedoke-McMaster hospitals under the care of the Palliative Care Team. They excluded from the group those who had only one contact with the team and of course they had no input to the exercise about the experience of patients who had no carers. They preferred this method of obtaining information to sending out a questionnaire which they saw as more impersonal and which might limit what respondents could say by the structure of the questions. For them the rationale was the importance of having consumer feedback in order to improve services. For those who attended the group it might provide information about the way they were coping with bereavement, and have some therapeutic benefit.

A key issue in audit is closing the audit loop – actually changing practice as a result of the audit if standards are not being met. This is the final hurdle where the process often falls down. Finlay (1993) discusses this problem and describes the procedure set up in her unit to carry out audit. She concludes that a mechanism which has been successful is to involve the whole team of nurses to evolve a new policy, with input from the nurse tutor, to create ownership throughout the team. She also emphasizes the important role of the chair of the audit meeting in helping the group to avoid destructive criticism and maintain momentum and cohesion.

8.5 CONCLUSION

Palliative care in the UK has come of age in the 1990s. It has the dignity of a chapter to itself in the Calman–Hine report *A Policy Framework for*

Commissioning Cancer Services (DoH, 1995b), the document which formed the basis for the direction of development of cancer services into the 21st century. The Executive Letter which takes further the guidance about purchasing palliative care in that report makes it clear that purchasers should not think of palliative care for cancer patients, but should extend it equally to other life-threatening diseases (NHS Executive, 1996). The NCHSPCS has established itself as a powerful voice for specialist palliative care services with the Department of Health and Government. Its influence is clear in the Executive letter cited above, which takes up the distinctions made by the Council between the palliative approach, palliative interventions and specialist palliative care, and in the consultation on the continuing care eligibility criteria.

Yet there are tensions and questions unanswered. Some challenge the National Council's definitions, asserting that much basic palliative care is carried out in the community by primary care teams with no specialist input and that this is more than simply using a palliative approach. The rapid development of specialist Hospital Support Teams has occurred with very little research on their effectiveness. Would it be more effective to put these resources into the community to prevent some of the hospital and hospice admissions which occur in the last week of life? Technological development is creating new opportunities for dramatic intervention in high-powered specialist medical centres, and at the other end of the spectrum making it possible to carry out many procedures locally and in the home, but with advice available from a specialist over a multimedia computer link. What impact will this have on the possibility of people dying at home? More exploration is needed of what specialists in palliative cancer care can offer to those dying from other diseases and what they need to learn to give appropriate care to those suffering from, say, heart disease or Alzheimer's disease in the final stages of the illness.

Beyond these service issues are the changes going on in attitudes to death and bereavement and in social relationships. The more individualistic approach to death, attitudes to risk taking, the increase in single person households and complex family structures – these are examples of the factors which will determine how palliative care develops in the 21st century. All these will have implications for the principles of open and sensitive communication, autonomy and choice, emphasizing quality of life, a holistic approach and a view of the unit of care encompassing the dying person and those who matter to them.

The experience of working close to dying people and those who care for them will continue to be challenging. Deschamps (1996) sets out the dangers. We must maintain contact with the 'irreducible anguish of humanity' but we must not become obsessed with it. A point comes when we must let the dying go and 'go back into our lives and heal the wound of loss'. However, this does not mean forgetting.

This book set out to provide a guide to good practice in the psychosocial aspects of palliative care, based on research and on what experienced practitioners are doing today. However, a major theme of the book has been how these principles underlying palliative care as it has developed so far may be followed through in practice. It is for the current generation of practitioners, teachers and researchers in palliative care to continue to test whether these principles are the right ones, and whether and how practice can deliver them for the benefit of dying people and their carers.

References

Abeles, M. (1991) Features of Judaism for carers when looking after Jewish patients. *Palliative Medicine*, **5**, 201–5.

Addington-Hall, J. and McCarthy, M. (1995) Dying from cancer: results of a national population-based investigation. *Palliative Medicine*, **9**, 295–305.

Addington-Hall, J., MacDonald, L.D., Anderson, H.R. and Freeling, P. (1991) Dying from cancer: the views of bereaved family and friends about the experiences of terminally ill patients. *Palliative Medicine*, **5**, 207–14.

Addington-Hall, J., MacDonald, L.D., Anderson, H.R., Chamberlain, J., Freeling, P., Bland, J. and Raftery, J. (1992) Randomised controlled trial of effects of co-ordinating care for terminally ill cancer patients. *British Medical Journal*, **305**, 1317–22.

Ahmedzai, S. (1993) Quality of life measurement in palliative care: philosophy, science or pontification? *Progress in Palliative Care*, **1**, 6–10.

Ajeman, I. (1993) The interdisciplinary team, in *Oxford Textbook of Palliative Medicine* (eds D. Doyle, G. Hanks and N. MacDonald), Oxford University Press, Oxford.

Alexander, D.A. (1993) Staff support groups: do they support and are they even groups? *Palliative Medicine*, **7**, 127–32.

Anderson, B.L. and Van Der Does, J. (1994) Surviving gynaecologic cancer and coping with sexual morbidity: an international problem. *International Journal of Gynaecologic Cancer*, **4**, 225–40.

Anthony, H. (1993) Some methodological problems in the assessment of complementary therapy, in *Clinical Research Methodology for Complementary Therapies* (eds G. Lewith and D. Aldridge), Hodder and Stoughton, London.

Aries, P. (1974) *Western Attitudes towards Death: from the middle ages to the present*, Johns Hopkins Press, Baltimore, MD.

Armstrong, D. (1987) Silence and truth in death and dying. *Social Science and Medicine*, **24**, 651–7.

Ashby, M. and Wakefield, M. (1993) Attitudes to some aspects of death and dying, living wills and substituted health care decision making in South Australia: public opinion survey for a parliamentary select committee. *Palliative Medicine*, **7**, 273–82.

Baider, L. and De-Nour, A.K. (1987) The meaning of disease: an exploratory study of Moslem Arab women after a mastectomy. *Journal of Psychosocial Oncology*, **4**, 1–13.

Barkwell, D.P. (1991) Ascribed meaning: a critical factor in coping and pain attenuation in patients with cancer-related pain. *Journal of Palliative Care*, **7**, 5–14.

Barnardo's (1994) *All About Me*, board game. Barnardo's, Barkingside, Essex.

Baulkwill, J. and Wood, C. (1994) Groupwork with bereaved children. *European Journal of Palliative Care*, **1**, 112–15.

Beck-Friis, B. and Strang, P. (1993) The organisation of hospital-based home care for terminally ill patients: the Motala model. *Palliative Medicine*, **7**, 93–100.

Belbin, R.M. (1981) *Management Teams*, Heinemann, London.

Benbow, S. and Quinn, A. (1990) Grief, dying and dementia. *Palliative Medicine*, **4**, 87–92.

Bendelow, G.A. and Williams, S.J. (1995) Sociological approaches to pain. *Progress in Palliative Care*, **3**, 169–80.

Bene, B. and Foxall, M.J. (1991) Death anxiety and job stress in hospice and medical-surgical nurses. *Hospice Journal*, **7**, 25–41.

Benner, P. (1984) *From Novice to Expert*, Addison Wesley, Reading, MA.

Berman, H., Cragg, C. and Kuenzig, L. (1988) Having a parent die of cancer. *Oncology Nursing Forum*, **15**, 159–63.

Bertman, S. (1991) *Facing Death: Images, Insights and Interventions*, Hemisphere, London.

Birdwhistell, R.L. (1970) *Kinesics and Context*, University of Pennsylvania Press, Philadelphia, PA.

Biswas, B. (1993) The medicalisation of dying: a nurse's view, in *The Future for Palliative Care* (ed. D. Clark), Open University Press, Buckingham.

Black, D. and Wood, D. (1989) Family therapy and life threatening illness in children or parents. *Palliative Medicine*, **3**, 113–8.

Blauner, R. (1966) Death and Social Structure. *Psychiatry*, **29**, 378–94.

Booth, K. (1995) Professional support and hospice nurses' blocking tactics during interviews. *Palliative Medicine*, **9**, 69.

Bowker, J. (1991) *The Meanings of Death*, Cambridge University Press, Cambridge.

Bowlby, J. (1969) *Attachment and Loss, Vol. 1, Attachment*, Basic Books, London.

Bram, P.J. and Katz, L.F. (1989) Study of burnout in nurses working in hospice and hospital oncology settings. *Oncology Nursing Forum*, **16**, 555–60.

Breitbart, W. and Passik, S. (1993) Psychiatric aspects of palliative care, in *Oxford Textbook of Palliative Medicine* (eds D. Doyle, G. Hanks and N. MacDonald), Oxford University Press, Oxford.

Brohn, P. (1987) *The Bristol Programme*, Century Hutchinson, London.

Brown, G. and Harris, T. (1978) *Social Origins of Depression: A Study of Psychiatric Disorder in Women*, Tavistock, London.

Buckman, R. (1988) *I Don't Know What to Say*, Macmillan, London.

Buckman, R. (1992) *How to Break Bad News: A Guide for Health-Care Professionals*, Papermac, London.

Buckman, R. (1993) Communication in palliative care: a practical guide, in *Oxford Textbook of Palliative Medicine* (eds D. Doyle, G. Hanks and N. Macdonald), Oxford University Press, Oxford.

Burroughs, A., Tyler, J., Moat, I. and Pye, S. (1992) Griefwork with children – workshop days at Pilgrim's Hospice in Canterbury. *Palliative Medicine*, **6**, 26–33.

Butler, R.N. (1963) The life review: an interpretation of reminiscence in the aged. *Psychiatry*, **26**, 65–73.

Calman, K. (1984) Quality of life in cancer patients. *Journal of Medical Ethics*, **10**, 124–7.

Cameron, J. and Parkes, C.M. (1983) Terminal care: evaluation of effects on surviving family of care before and after bereavement. *Postgraduate Medicine Journal*, **59**, 73–8.

Cancer Relief Macmillan Fund (1994) *Organisational Audit for Specialist Palliative Care Services*, Cancer Relief Macmillan Fund, London.

Carter, P. (1994) *The Thursday Group*. Hospice Information Service, October 1994, p. 5.

Cartwright, A., Hockey, L. and Anderson, J.A. (1973) *Life before Death*, Routledge and Kegan Paul, London.

Cartwright, A. and Seale. C. (1990) *The Natural History of a Survey: An Account of the Methodological Issues Encountered in a Study of Life Before Death*, King Edward's Hospital Fund for London, London.

Cartwright, A. and Seale, C. (1994) *The Year before Death*, Avebury, Aldershot.

Cassileth, B., Lush, E.J., Strouse, T.B. and Bodenheimer, B.J. (1984) Contemporary unorthodox treatments in cancer medicine: a study of patients, treatments and practitioners. *Annals of Internal Medicine*, **101**, 105–12.

Clark, D. (1982) *Between Pulpit and Pew*, Cambridge University Press, Cambridge.

Clark, D. (1991) Contradictions in the development of new hospices: a case study. *Social Science and Medicine*, **33**, 995–1004.

Clarke, M., Finlay, I. and Campbell, I. (1991) Cultural boundaries in care. *Palliative Medicine*, **5**, 63–5.

Cocker, K.I., Bell, D.R. and Kidman, A. (1994) Cognitive behaviour therapy with advanced breast cancer patients. *Psycho-oncology*, **3**, 233–7.

Cohen, P. (1996) Death duties. *Community Care*, 18–24 January, **11–12**.

Cole, R.M. (1993) Communicating with people who request euthanasia. *Palliative Medicine*, **7**, 139–43.

Coles, C. (1996) Undergraduate education and palliative care. *Palliative Medicine*, **10**, 93–8.

Connell, C. (1992) Art therapy as part of a palliative care programme. *Palliative Medicine*, **6**, 18–25.

Copp, G. and Dunn, V. (1993) Frequent and difficult problems perceived by nurses caring for the dying in community, hospice and acute care settings. *Palliative Medicine*, **7**, 19–25.

Corner, J. (1996) Is there a research paradigm for palliative care? *Palliative Medicine*, **10**, 201–8.

Corner, J., Cawley, N. and Hildebrand, S. (1995) An evaluation of the use of massage and essential oils on the well-being of cancer patients. *International Journal of Cancer Nursing*, **1**, 67–73.

Corr, C. (1991–92) A task-based approach to dying. *Omega*, **24**, 81–94.

Council of Europe (1995) *Multiprofessional education of health personnel,* Council of Europe Press, Strasbourg.

Davies, B. and Oberle, K. (1990) Dimensions of the supportive role of the nurse in palliative care. *Oncology Nursing Forum,* **17,** 87–94.

Deschamps, D. (1996) Supporting the dying in myth and reality. *European Journal of Palliative Care,* **3,** 72–4.

DHSS (1976) *Prevention and Health: Everybody's Business,* HMSO, London.

DHSS (1980) *Report of the Working Group on Terminal Care,* HMSO, London.

Dittman-Kohli, F. (1990) The construction of meaning in old age: possibilities and constraints. *Ageing and Society,* **10,** 270–94.

DoH (1989) *Caring for People: Community Care in the Next Decade and Beyond,* Cmd 849, HMSO, London.

DoH (1995a) *NHS Responsibilities for Meeting Continuing Care Needs,* HSG(95)8: LAC(95)5, Department of Health, London.

DoH (1995b) *A Policy Framework for Commissioning Cancer Services,* A Report by the Expert Advisory Group on Cancer to the Chief Medical Officers of England and Wales, Department of Health, London.

Douglas, C. (1991) For all the saints. *British Medical Journal,* **304,** 579.

Downer, S.M., Cody, M.M., McCluskey, P., Wilson, P.D., Arnott, S., Lister, T.A. and Slevin, M. (1994) Pursuit and practice of complementary therapies by cancer patients receiving conventional treatment. *British Medical Journal,* **309,** 86–9.

Doyle, D. (1980) Domiciliary terminal care. *Practitioner,* **224,** 575–82.

Doyle, D. (1993a) Specialist Palliative Care Services Defined, in *Needs Assessment for Hospice and Specialist Palliative Care Services: from philosophy to contracts,* Occasional Paper No. 4, National Council for Hospice and Specialist Palliative Care Services, London.

Doyle, D. (1993b) Palliative Medicine – a time for definition? *Palliative Medicine,* **7,** 253–5.

Dunlop, R., Davies, R.J. and Hockley, J. (1989) Preferred versus actual place of death. *Palliative Medicine,* **3,** 197–201.

Dunne, J. and Jenkins, L. (1991) *Stress and Coping Strategies in Macmillan Nurses,* Cancer Relief Macmillan Fund, London.

Dunphy, K., Finlay, I., Rathbone, G., Gilbert, J. and Hicks, F. (1995) Rehydration in palliative and terminal care – if not, why not? *Palliative Medicine,* **9,** 221–8.

Earnshaw-Smith, E. and Yorkstone, P. (1986) *Setting up and running a bereavement service,* St Christopher's Hospice, London.

Eastleigh Carers' Group (1992) *What We Have to Say...* A report from the Eastleigh Carers' Group.

Egan, G. (1994) *The Skilled Helper,* 5th edn, Brooks Cole, Pacific Grove, CA.

Eisenbruch, M. (1984) Cross-cultural aspects of bereavement. 1: A conceptual framework for comparative analysis. *Culture, Medicine and Psychiatry,* **8,** 283–309.

Ellison, C.W. (1982) Spiritual well-being: conceptualisation and measurement. *Journal of Psychology and Theology,* **11,** 330–40.

Engel, G.L. (1961) Is grief a disease? *Psychosomatic Medicine,* **23,** 18–22.

Erikson, E.H. (1965) *Childhood and Society,* Hogarth, London.

European Association for Palliative Care (1989) Newsletter, Spring, Milan.

Evans, A.J. (1994) Anticipatory grief: a theoretical challenge. *Palliative Medicine*, **8**, 159–65.

Eve, A.M. and Smith, A. (1994) Palliative care services in Britain and Ireland – update 1991. *Palliative Medicine*, **8**, 19–27.

Fallowfield, L. (1992) The quality of life: sexual function and body image following cancer therapy. *Cancer Topics*, **9**, 20–1.

Faulkner, A., Higginson, I., Egerton, H., Power, M., Sykes, N. and Wilkes, E. (1993) *Hospice Day Care – A Qualitative Study*, Help the Hospices, London.

Faull, C., Johnson, I.S. and Butler, T.J. (1994) The hospital anxiety and depression (HAD) scale: its validity in patients with terminal malignant disease. *Palliative Medicine*, **8**, 69.

Field, D., Douglas, C., Jagger, C. and Dand, P. (1995) Terminal illness: views of lay patients and their carers. *Palliative Medicine*, **9**, 45–54.

Field, D. and Johnson, I. (1993) Satisfaction and change: a survey of volunteers in a hospice organisation. *Social Science and Medicine*, **36**, 1625–33.

Finlay, I. (1993) Audit experience: views of a hospice director, in *Clinical Audit in Palliative Care* (ed. I. Higginson), Radcliffe Medical Press, Oxford.

Firth, P. and Anderson, P. (1994) Teamwork with families facing bereavement. *European Journal of Palliative Care*, **1**, 157–61.

Firth, S. (1993) Cultural issues in terminal care, in *The Future for Palliative Care* (ed. D. Clark), Open University Press, Buckingham.

Fish, W.C. (1986) Differences of grief intensity of bereaved parents, in *Parental Loss of a Child* (ed. T. Rando), Research Press, Champaign, IL.

Fisher, R. (1991) Introduction: Palliative care – a rediscovery, in *Palliative Care for People with Cancer* (eds J. Penson and R. Fisher), Edward Arnold, London.

Foley, F.J., Flannery, J., Graydon, D., Flintoft, G. and Cook, D. (1995) AIDS palliative care – challenging the palliative paradigm. *Journal of Palliative Care*, **11**, 19–22.

Ford, G. (1993) The development of palliative care services, in *The Oxford Textbook of Palliative Medicine* (eds D. Doyle, G. Hanks and N. Macdonald), Oxford University Press, Oxford.

Foulstone, S., Harvey, B., Wright, J., Jay, M., Owen, F. and Cole, R. (1993) Bereavement support: evaluation of a palliative care memorial service. *Palliative Medicine*, **7**, 307–11.

Frampton, D. (1993) Creative arts and literature, in *Oxford Textbook of Palliative Medicine* (eds D. Doyle, G. Hanks and N. MacDonald), Oxford University Press, Oxford.

Frank, J. (1995) *Couldn't Care More: A Study of Young Carers and their Needs*, The Children's Society, London.

Frankl, V. (1987) *Man's Search for Meaning*, Hodder and Stoughton, London.

Freedman, T. (1994) Social and cultural dimensions of hair loss in women treated for breast cancer. *Cancer Nursing*, **17**, 334–41.

Freud, S. (1917) Mourning and melancholia, in *Standard Edition of the Complete Psychological Works of Sigmund Freud*, Vol. 14 (ed. J. Strachey), Hogarth, London.

Froggatt, K. (1995) *Order in disorder: rites of passage in the hospice culture*, paper given at The Second International Conference of Death and Dying, University of Sussex, Brighton, September.

Gerber, I., Rusalem, R., Hannon, N., Battin, D. and Arkin, A. (1975) Anticipatory grief and aged widows and widowers. *Journal of Gerontology*, **30**, 225–9.

Gersie, A. (1991) *Storymaking in Bereavement: Dragons Fight in the Meadow*, Jessica Kingsley, London.

Gibbs, G. (1995) Nurses in private nursing homes: a study of their knowledge and attitudes to pain management in palliative care. *Palliative Medicine*, **9**, 245–53.

Gilley, J. (1988) Intimacy and terminal care. *Journal of the Royal College of General Practitioners*, **38**, 121–2.

Glaser, B. and Strauss, A. (1965) *Awareness of Dying*, Aldine, Chicago, IL.

Gomez-Batiste, X., Borras, J., Fontanels, M., Stjernsward, J. and Trias, X. (1992) Palliative care in Catalonia 1990–95. *Palliative Medicine*, **6**, 321–7.

Gorer, G. (1965) *Death, Grief and Mourning in Contemporary Britain*, Cresset, London.

Haight, B., Coleman, P. and Lord, K. (1995) The linchpins of successful life review: structure, evaluation and individuality, in *The Art and Science of Reminiscing: theory, research, methods and application* (eds B. Haight and J. Webster), Taylor and Francis, Washington, DC.

Hall, J. and Kirschling, J. (1990) A conceptual framework for caring for families of hospice patients, in *Family-Based Palliative Care* (ed. J. Kirschling), Haworth, New York.

Hampe, S.O. (1975) Needs of the grieving spouse in hospital. *Nursing Research*, **24**, 113–19.

Hartley, S. (1996) *Gender differences in parental bereavement following childhood cancer: the impact of employment on the recovery process*, unpublished M.Sc. dissertation, University of Southampton.

Heaven, C. and Maguire, P. (1995) Disclosure and identification of concerns in hospices. *Palliative Medicine*, **9**, 70.

Heegard, M. (1991) *When Someone has a Very Serious Illness*, Woodland, Minneapolis, MN.

Helman, C.G. (1994) *Culture, Health and Illness*, 3rd edn, Butterworth-Heinemann, Oxford.

Hemmings, P. (1994) Working with children facing bereavement as individuals. *European Journal of Palliative Care*, **1**, 72–7.

Herth, K. (1989) The relationship between level of hope and level of coping response and other variables in patients with cancer. *Oncology Nursing Forum*, **16**, 67–72.

Herth, K. (1990) Fostering hope in terminally ill people. *Journal of Advanced Nursing*, **15**, 1250–9.

Heyse-Moore, L.H. and Johnson, V.E. (1987) Can doctors accurately predict the life expectancy of patients with terminal cancer? *Palliative Medicine*, **1**, 165–6.

Higginson, I. (1992) *Quality, Standards, Organisational and Clinical Audit for Hospice and Palliative Care Services*. Occasional Paper No. 2, National Council for Hospice and Specialist Palliative Care Services, London.

Higginson, I. (1993a) Palliative care: a review of past changes and future trends. *Journal of Public Health Medicine*, **15**, 3–8.

Higginson, I. (ed.) (1993b) *Clinical Audit in Palliative Care*, Radcliffe Medical Press, Oxford.

Higginson, I. and McCarthy, M. (1993) Validity of the support team assessment schedule: do staffs' ratings reflect those made by patients or their families? *Palliative Medicine*, **7**, 219–28.

Higginson, I., Wade, A. and McCarthy, M. (1992) Effectiveness of two palliative support teams. *Journal of Public Health Medicine*, **1**, 50–6.

Higginson, I., Webb, D. and Lessof, L. (1994) Reducing hospital beds for patients with advanced cancer. *Lancet*, **344**, 409.

Hildebrand, J. (1989) Working with a bereaved family: focusing on prevention not pathology. *Palliative Medicine*, **3**, 105–11.

Hillier, E.R. (1983) Terminal care in the UK, in *Hospice Care: Principles and Practice* (eds C. Corr and D. Corr), Faber and Faber, London.

Hinton, J. (1963) The physical and mental distress of the dying. *Quarterly Journal of Medicine*, **32**, 1–22.

Hinton, J. (1967) *Dying*, Penguin, Harmondsworth.

Hinton, J. (1994a) Which patients with terminal cancer are admitted from home care? *Palliative Medicine*, **8**, 197–210.

Hinton, J. (1994b) Can home care maintain an acceptable quality of life for patients with terminal cancer and their relatives? *Palliative Medicine*, **8**, 183–96.

Hinton, J. (1996) Services given and help perceived during home care for terminal cancer. *Palliative Medicine*, **10**, 125–34.

Hogbin, B. and Fallowfield, L. (1989) Getting it taped: the 'bad news' consultation with cancer patients. *British Journal of Hospital Medicine*, **4**, 330–3.

Honeybun, J., Johnston, M. and Tookman, A. (1992) The impact of a death on fellow hospice patients. *British Journal of Medical Psychology*, **65**, 67–72.

Hopkins, A. (1993) Clinical Audit in Palliative Care: a critical appraisal, in *Clinical Audit in Palliative Care* (ed. I. Higginson), Radcliffe Medical Press, Oxford.

Hospice Information Bulletin (1991) *Hospice – What People Think*, Hospice Information Bulletin No. 11, St Christopher's Hospice, London.

Hull, M. (1990) Sources of stress for hospice care-giving families, in *Family-based Palliative Care* (ed. J. Kirschling), Howarth, New York.

Hunt, M. (1992) 'Scripts' for dying at home – displayed in nurses' patients' and relatives talk. *Journal of Advanced Nursing*, **17**, 1297–302.

Hunt, R., Maddocks, I., Roach, D. and McLeod, A. (1991) The incidence of requests for a quicker terminal course. *Palliative Medicine*, **9**, 167–8.

Hunt, R. and McCaul, K. (1996) A population based study of the coverage of cancer patients by hospice services. *Palliative Medicine*, **10**, 5–12.

Hutchinson, S. (1995) Evaluation of bereavement anniversary cards. *Journal of Palliative Care*, **11**, 32–4.

Ignatieff, M. (1990) *The Needs of Strangers,* Hogarth, London.

Iles, P. and Auluck, R. (1990) Team building, inter-agency team development and social work practice. *British Journal of Social Work*, **20**, 151–64.

Illich, I. (1977) *The Limits to Medicine*, Penguin, Harmondsworth.

Information Exchange (1996) School's children share their sadness. *Information Exchange*, May.

Ingleton, C. and Faulkner, A. (1994) *Quality Assurance in Palliative Care: A Review of the Literature*, Occasional Paper No. 14, Trent Palliative Care Centre, Sheffield.

Irwin, M. and Pike, J. (1993) Bereavement, depressive symptoms and immune function, in *Handbook of Bereavement: Theory, Research and Intervention* (eds

M.S. Stroebe, W. Stroebe and R.O. Hansson), University of Cambridge Press, Cambridge.

Jackson, L. (1990) Team Building, in *Hospice and Palliative Care: An Interdisciplinary Approach* (ed. C. Saunders), Edward Arnold, London.

James, N. (1988) A family and a team – nurses' roles in in-patient terminal care, in *A Safer Death: Multidisciplinary Aspects of Terminal Care* (eds A. Gilmore and S. Gilmore), Plenum Press, New York.

James, N. and Field, D. (1992) The routinisation of hospice: charisma and bureaucratisation. *Social Science and Medicine,* **14**, 488–509.

Jarrett, N. and Payne, S. (1995) A selective review of the literature on nurse-patient communication – has the patient's contribution been neglected? *Journal of Advanced Nursing,* **22**, 72–8.

Jenkins, H. (1989) The family and loss: a systems framework. *Palliative Medicine,* **3**, 97–104.

Jones, K., Johnston, M. and Speck, P. (1989) Despair felt by the patient and the professional carer: a case study of the use of cognitive behavioural methods. *Palliative Medicine,* **3**, 39–46.

Jones, R.V.H. (1992) Teamwork in primary care: how much do we know about it? *Journal of Interprofessional Care,* **6**, 25–9.

Jones, R.V.H. (1993) Teams and terminal cancer at home: do patients and carers benefit? *Journal of Interprofessional Care,* **7**, 239–44.

Kane, B. (1979) Children's concepts of death. *Journal of Genetic Psychology,* **4**, 15–17.

Karl, G.T. (1987) A new look at grief. *Journal of Advanced Nursing,* **12**, 641–5.

Kastenbaum, R. (1975) Is death a life-crisis? in *Lifespan Developmental Psychology: Normative Life Crises* (eds N. Datan and L. Ginsberg), Academic Press, New York.

Kaye, P. (1989) *Notes on Symptom Control in Hospice and Palliative Care*, Hospice Education Institute, Essex, CT.

Kearney, M. (1992a) Palliative medicine: just another specialty? *Palliative Medicine,* **6**, 39–46.

Kearney, M. (1992b) Imagework in a case of intractable pain. *Palliative Medicine,* **6**, 152–7.

Kennedy, I. (1981) *The Unmasking of Medicine*, Allen and Unwin, London.

Kim, K. and Jacobs, S. (1993) Neuroendocrine changes following bereavement, in *Handbook of Bereavement: Theory, Research and Intervention* (eds M.S. Stroebe, W. Stroebe and R.O. Hansson), University of Cambridge Press, Cambridge.

King, M., Speck, P. and Thomas, A. (1994) Spiritual and religious beliefs in acute illness – is this a feasible area for study? *Social Science and Medicine,* **38**, 631–6.

Kirschling, J., Tilden, V.P. and Butterfield, P.G. (1990) Social support: the experience of hospice family caregivers, in *Family-Based Palliative Care* (ed. J. Kirschling), Howarth Press, New York.

Kissane, D.W., Bloch, S., Ivon Burns, W., McKenzies, D. and Posterino, M. (1994) Psychological morbidity in the families of cancer patients with cancer. *Psychooncology,* **3**, 47–56.

Kissane, D., Finlay, I. and George, R. (1996) Euthanasia in Australia. *Progress in Palliative Care,* **4**, 71–3.

Knaus, W.A., Draper, E.A., Wagner, D.P. and Zimmerman, J.E. (1986) An evaluation of outcome from intensive care in major medical centres. *Annals of Internal Medicine*, **104**, 410–19.

Kuebler-Ross, E. (1970) *On Death and Dying*, Tavistock, London.

Lamerton, R. (1973) *Care of the Dying*, Priory Press, Sussex.

Lanceley, A. (1995) Emotional disclosure between cancer patients and nurses, in *Nursing Research in Cancer Care* (eds A. Richardson and J. Wilson-Barnett), Scutari Press, London.

Lansdown, R. and Benjamin, G. (1985) The development of the concept of death in children aged 5 to 9. *Child Care Health Development*, **11**, 13–20.

Lauer, M., Mulhern, R., Bohne, H. and Camitta, B. (1985) Children's perceptions of their sibling's death: the precursors of differential adjustment. *Cancer Nursing*, **8**, 21–7.

Leriche, R. (1939) *The Surgery of Pain*, Ballière, Tindall and Cox, London.

Lester, J. (1995) *Life review with the terminally ill*, unpublished M.Sc. dissertation, University of Southampton.

Levin, E., Moriarty, J. and Gorbacy, P. (1994) *Better for the Break*, HMSO, London.

Lewis, C.S. (1961) *A Grief Observed*, Faber, London.

Lichter, I. (1993) Biography as therapy. *Palliative Medicine*, **7**, 133–7.

Lieberman, M.A. (1993) Bereavement self-help groups, in *Handbook of Bereavement: Theory, Research and Intervention* (eds M.S. Stroebe, W. Stroebe and R.O. Hansson), University of Cambridge Press, Cambridge.

Lloyd-Williams, M. (1996) A survey of palliative care given to patients with end-stage dementia. Paper given at the Palliative Care Research Forum, Durham UK 8–9 November 1995. Abstract published in *Palliative Medicine*, **10**, 63.

Lonsdale, S., Webb, A. and Briggs, T. (eds) (1980) *Teamwork in the Personal Social Services*, Croom Helm, London.

Lund, D.A., Dimond, M.F., Caserta, M.S., Johnson, R.J., Poulton, J.L. and Connelly, J.R. (1985–86) Identifying elderly with coping difficulties after 2 years of bereavement. *Omega*, **16**, 213–23.

Lunn, L. (1993) Spiritual concerns in palliative care, in *The Management of Terminal Malignant Disease* (eds C. Saunders and N. Sykes), Edward Arnold, London.

Lunt, B., Neale, C. and Clifford, C. (1985) *A comparison of hospice and hospital care for terminally ill cancer patients and their families*. Accompanying Paper B. Unpublished report of DHSS funded research.

Lunt, B. and Yardley, J. (1988) *Home Care Teams and Hospital Support Teams for the Terminally Ill*. Cancer Relief Macmillan Fund, London.

Maccabee, J. (1994) The effect of transfer from a palliative care unit to a nursing home. *Palliative Medicine*, **8**, 211–14.

Mackay, M. (1993) *Dementia and Bereavement*, Dementia Services Development Centre, University of Stirling.

Macleod, J. (1996) Symptom management in transcultural nursing. *European Journal of Palliative Care*, **2**, 124–6.

Maddison, D. and Walker, W.L. (1967) Factors affecting the outcome of conjugal bereavement. *British Journal of Psychiatry*, **113**, 1057–67.

Maddocks, I. (1993) 'Good palliative care' orders. *Palliative Medicine*, **7**, 35–7.

Maguire, P. (1985) Barriers to psychological care of the dying. *British Medical Journal*, **291**, 1711–13.

Maguire, P. and Buckman, R. (1985) *Why Won't They Talk to Me?* Videotape Linkward Productions, Shepperton, Middlesex.

Maguire, P. and Faulkner, A. (1988) How to do it. Communicate with cancer patients and their relatives. 1. Handling bad news and difficult questions. 2. Handling collusion, uncertainty and denial. *British Medical Journal*, **297**, 907–9, 972–4.

Maguire, P. (1995) Psychosocial interventions to reduce affective disorders in cancer patients: research priorities. *Psycho-oncology*, **4**, 113–19.

Martin, J. (1989) Doctor's mask on pain, in *Death, Dying and Bereavement* (eds D. Dickenson and M Johnson), Sage, London.

Mathers, P. (1995) Learning to cope with the stress of palliative care, in *Palliative Care for People with Cancer*, 2nd edn (eds J. Penson and R. Fisher), Edward Arnold, London.

Mawson, D., Marks, I.M., Ramm, L. and Stern, R.S. (1981) Guided mourning for morbid grief: a controlled study. *British Journal of Psychiatry*, **138**, 185–93.

Mayo, S. (1996) Symbol, metaphor and story: the function of group art therapy in palliative care. *Palliative Medicine*, **10**, 209–16.

McGee, R. (1984) Hope: a factor influencing crisis resolution. *Advances in Nursing Science*, July, 34–44.

McIllmurray, M.B., Gorst, D.W., Shand, W.S., Crimmin, M. and Thomas, J.A. (1992) Sculptors in residence: report of a Lancaster project. *Palliative Medicine*, **6**, 34–8.

McKee, E. (1993) Audit experience: a nurse manager in home care, in *Clinical Audit in Palliative Care* (ed. I. Higginson), Radcliffe Medical Press, Oxford.

Mead, M. (1953) *Cultural Patterns and Technical Change*, UNESCO, Paris.

Mesler, M. (1994–95) The philosophy and practice of patient control in hospice: the dynamics of autonomy versus paternalism. *Omega*, **30**, 173–89.

Middleton, W., Raphael, B., Martinek, N. and Misso, V. (1993) Pathological grief reactions, in *Handbook of Bereavement: Theory, Research and Intervention* (eds M.S. Stroebe, W. Stroebe and R.O. Hansson), Cambridge University Press, Cambridge.

Mills, M., Davies, H.T.O. and Macrae, W.A. (1994) Care of dying patients in hospital. *British Medical Journal*, **309**, 583–6.

Minuchin, S. (1974) *Families and Family Therapy*, Tavistock, London.

Monroe, B. (1993a) Psychosocial dimension of palliation, in *The Management of Terminal Malignant Disease* (eds C. Saunders and N. Sykes), Edward Arnold, London.

Monroe, B. (1993b) The cost to the professional carer, in *The Management of Terminal Malignant Disease* (eds C. Saunders and N. Sykes), Edward Arnold, London.

Moorey, S. and Greer, S. (1989) *Psychological Therapy for Cancer Patients*, Heinemann Medical Books, Oxford.

Mulder, C.L., Van der Pompe, G., Spiegel, D., Antoni, M.H. and De Vries, M. (1992) Do psychosocial factors influence the course of breast cancer? A review of the literature, methodological problems and future directions. *Psycho-oncology*, **1**, 155–67.

Munnichs, J. (1987) *Finitude and Dying: Contributions to Gerontological and Thanatological Research*, The Southampton Papers, Southampton University 1987.

Munro, S. and Mount, B. (1978) Music therapy in palliative care. *Canadian Medical Association Journal*, **119**, 3–8.

NAHAT (1990) *Care of the Dying: District Health Authority Support to Hospices and Trusts, an Update*, National Association of Health Authorities and Trusts, Birmingham.

Nash, A. (1993) Reasons for referral to a palliative nursing team. *Journal of Advanced Nursing*, **18**, 707–13.

Nash, A. and Hoy, A. (1993) Terminal care in the community – an evaluation of residential workshops. *Palliative Medicine*, **7**, 5–17.

National Council for Hospice and Specialist Palliative Care Services (1995a) *Specialist Palliative Care: A Statement of Definitions*, Occasional Paper No. 8, London, October.

National Council for Hospice and Specialist Palliative Care. (1995b) *Opening Doors: Improving Access to Hospice and Specialist Palliative Care Services by Members of the Black and Ethnic Minority Communities*, Occasional Paper No. 7, London, January.

Neale, C. (1989) *Getting on with Living*, Graves Medical Audiovisual Library No. 89-4, Chelmsford. Essex.

Neale, B. (1991) *Informal Palliative Care: A Review of Research on Needs, Standards and Service Evaluation*, Occasional Paper No. 3, Trent Palliative Care Centre, Sheffield.

Ness, D.E. and Ende, J. (1994) Denial in the medical interview: recognition and management. *Journal of the American Medical Association*, **272**, 1777–81.

Neuberger, J. (1987) *Caring for Dying People of Different Faiths*, Austen Cornish and the Lisa Sainsbury Foundation.

Neuberger, J (1993) Cultural issues in palliative care, in *Oxford Textbook of Palliative Medicine* (eds D. Doyle, G Hanks and N. Macdonald), Oxford University Press, London.

NHS Executive (1996) EL(96)85. *A Policy Framework for Commissioning Cancer Services: Palliative Care Services.* London.

Oken, D. (1961) What to tell cancer patients: a study of medical attitudes. *Journal of the American Medical Association*, **175**, 1120–8.

Oliviere, D. (1993) Cross-cultural principles of care, in *The Management of Terminal Malignant Disease* (eds C. Saunders and N Sykes), Edward Arnold, London.

Oswin, M. (1993) The grief that does not speak, in *Death, Dying and Bereavement* (eds D. Dickenson and M. Johnson), Sage, London.

Owen, C., Tennant, C., Levi, J. and Jones, M. (1992) Suicide and euthanasia: attitudes in the context of cancer. *Psycho-oncology*, **1**, 79–88.

Parkes, C.M. (1971) Psychosocial transitions: a field for study. *Social Science and Medicine*, **5**, 101–15.

Parkes, C.M. (1975) Unexpected and untimely bereavement: a statistical study of young Boston widows and widowers, in *Bereavement: its psychological aspects* (eds B. Schoenberg, I. Gerber, A. Wiener, D. Kutscher, D. Peretz and A. Cam), Columbia University Press, New York.

Parkes, C.M. (1982) How should a counsellor respond to the threat of suicide after bereavement. *Bereavement Care*, **1**, 5.

Parkes, C.M. (1986) *Bereavement: Studies of Grief in Adult Life*, 2nd edn, Penguin, Harmondsworth.

Parkes, C.M. (1990) Risk factors in bereavement: implications for the prevention and treatment of pathologic grief. *Psychiatric Annals*, **20**, 308–13.

Parkes, C.M. and Weiss, R.S. (1983) *Recovery from Bereavement*, Basic Books, New York.

Parkes, C.M., Stevenson-Hinde, J. and Marris, P. (1991) *Attachment across the Life Cycle*, Routledge, London.

Payne, S. and Relf, M. (1994) The assessment of need for bereavement follow-up in palliative and hospice care. *Palliative Medicine*, **8**, 291–7.

Penn, K. (1994) Patient advocacy in palliative care. *British Journal of Nursing*, **3**, 40–2.

Pennells, M. and Kitchener, S. (1990) Holding back the nightmares. *Social Work Today*, 1 March, 14–15.

Penson, J. (1995) Complementary therapies, in *Palliative Care for People with Cancer*, 2nd edn (eds J. Penson and R. Fisher), Edward Arnold, London.

Pickrel, J. (1989) Tell me your story: using life review in counselling the terminally ill. *Death Studies*, **13**, 127–35.

Pitcher, P. (1996) *The personal bereavement experience of nurses working in palliative care*, unpublished MSc dissertation, University of Southampton.

Raftery, J., Addington-Hall, J., MacDonald, L.R., Anderson, H.R., Bland, J., Chamberlain, J. and Freeling, P. (1996) A randomised controlled trial of the cost-effectiveness of a district co-ordinating service for terminally ill cancer patients. *Palliative Medicine*, **10**, 151–61.

Ramsay, R.W. (1977) Behavioral approaches to bereavement. *Behaviour Research and Therapy*, **15**, 131–5.

Randall, F. and Downie, R.S. (1996) *Palliative Care Ethics: A Good Companion*, Oxford Medical Publications/Oxford University Press, Oxford.

Raphael, B. (1983) *The Anatomy of Bereavement*, Basic Books, New York.

Rathbone, G., Horsley, S. and Goacher, J. (1994) A self-evaluated assessment for seriously ill hospice patients. *Palliative Medicine*, **8**, 29–34.

Registrar General (1969) *The Registrar General's Statistical Review of England and Wales for the Year 1969*, HMSO, London.

Reimer, J.C., Davies, B. and Martens, N. (1991) The nurse's role in helping families through the transition of 'fading away'. *Cancer Nursing*, **14**, 321–7.

Relf, M. (1997) *How effective are volunteers in providing bereavement care?*, in Proceedings of the Fourth Congress of the European Association for Palliative Care, Barcelona, 6–9 December 1995.

Relf, M. and Couldrick, A. (1988) Bereavement Support: the relationship between professionals and volunteers, in *A Safer Death: Multidisciplinary Aspects of Terminal Care* (eds A. Gilmore and S. Gilmore), Plenum Press, New York.

Robbins, M., Jackson, P., Brooks, J. and Frankel, S. (1995) Framing the sample in palliative care research: reflections from one district. Paper presented at the Palliative Care Research Forum, Durham, 8–9 November 1995. Abstract published in *Palliative Medicine*, **10**, 55.

Roisin, D., Laval, G. and Lelut, B. (1994) Interdisciplinary activity in a mobile palliative care team. *European Journal of Palliative Care*, **1**, 132–5.

Rosenblatt, P.C. (1993) Grief: the social context of private feelings, in *Handbook of Bereavement: Theory, Research and Intervention* (eds M.S. Stroebe, W. Stroebe and R.O. Hansson), University of Cambridge Press, Cambridge.

Ross, D.M., Petcet, J., Mediros, C., Walsh-Burke, K. and Rieker, P. (1992) Differences between nurses and physicians' approach to denial in oncology. *Cancer Nursing*, **15**, 422–8.

Rutter, M. (1966) *Children of Sick Parents*, Oxford University Press, London.

Sanders, C. (1993) Risk factors in bereavement, in *Handbook of Bereavement: Theory, Research and Intervention* (eds M.S. Stroebe, W. Stroebe and R.O. Hansson), University of Cambridge Press, Cambridge.

Saunders, C. (1993) Introduction – history and challenge, in *The Management of Terminal Malignant Disease*, 3rd edn (eds C. Saunders and N. Sykes), Hodder and Stoughton, London.

Saunders, C., Summers, D. and Teller, N. (1981) *Hospice – The Living Idea*, Edward Arnold, London.

Seale, C. (1991) Death from cancer and death from other causes: the relevance of the hospice approach. *Palliative Medicine*, **5**, 12–19.

Seale, C. and Addington-Hall, J. (1994) Euthanasia: why people want to die earlier. *Social Science and Medicine*, **39**, 647–54.

Seale, C. and Cartwright, A. (1994) *The Year before Death*, Avebury, Aldershot.

Seligman, P. (1975) *Helplessness: on Depression, Development and Death*, Freeman, San Francisco, CA.

Sheldon, F. (1995) Will the doors open? Multicultural issues in palliative care. *Palliative Medicine*, **9**, 89–90.

Sheldon, F. and Smith, P. (1996) The life so short, the craft so hard to learn: a model for post-basic education. *Palliative Medicine*, **10**, 93–8.

Shneidman, E.S. (1975) *Deaths of Man*, Quadrangle, New York.

Silverman, P. and Worden, J.W. (1993) Children's reactions to the death of a parent, in *Handbook of Bereavement: Theory, Research and Intervention* (eds M.S. Stroebe, W. Stroebe and R.O. Hansson), University of Cambridge Press, Cambridge.

SMAC/SNMAC (1992) *The Principles and Provision of Palliative Care. Joint Report of the Standing Medical Advisory Committee and Standing Nursing and Midwifery Advisory Committee*, HMSO, London.

Small, N. (1993) HIV/AIDS: Lessons for Policy and Practice, in *The Future for Palliative Care* (ed. D. Clark), Open University Press, Buckingham.

Smith, A, and Eve, A.M. (1994) Palliative care services in Britain and Ireland – update 1991. *Palliative Medicine*, **8**, 19–27.

Smith, N. and Regnard, C. (1993) Managing family problems in advanced disease – a flow diagram. *Palliative Medicine*, **7**, 47–58.

Speck, P. (1993) Spiritual issues in palliative care, in *The Oxford Textbook of Palliative Medicine* (eds D. Doyle, G. Hanks and N. Macdonald), Oxford University Press, Oxford.

Spiegel, D., Bloom, J., Kraemer, H.C. and Gotheil, E. (1989) Effect of psychosocial treatment on survival of patients with metastatic breast cancer. *Lancet*, **ii**, 888–91.

Spiller, J.A. and Alexander, D.A. (1993) Domiciliary care: views of terminally ill patients and their families. *Palliative Medicine*, **7**, 109–15.

Stedeford, A. (1984*) Facing Death: Patients, Families and Professionals*, Heinemann Medical Books, Oxford.

Stern, K. (1993) Living wills in English law. *Palliative Medicine*, **7**, 283–8.

Stroebe, M. (1992–93) Coping with bereavement: a review of the griefwork hypothesis. *Omega*, **26**, 19–42.

Stroebe, M.S. (1994) *Helping the bereaved to come to terms with loss: what does bereavement research have to offer?* Keynote address at the Conference on Bereavement and Counselling, St George's Hospital Medical School, 25 March.

Stroebe, M.S. and Stroebe, W. (1993) The mortality of bereavement, in *Handbook of Bereavement: Theory, Research and Intervention* (eds M.S. Stroebe, W. Stroebe and R.O. Hansson), University of Cambridge Press, Cambridge.

Styles, B. (1994) Viol bodies. *Health Service Journal*, 3 February, 30–2.

Stylianos, S.K. and Vachon, M. (1993) Social support in bereavement, in *Handbook of Bereavement: Theory, Research and Intervention* (eds M.S. Stroebe, W. Stroebe and R.O Hansson), University of Cambridge, Cambridge.

Sykes, N., Pearson, S. and Chell, S. (1992) Quality of care: the carer's perspective. *Palliative Medicine*, **6**, 227–36.

Taylor, H. (1983) *The Hospice Movement in Britain: Its Role and its Future*, Centre for Policy on Ageing, London.

The Life that's Left. (1977) Film and Video Library CTVC, Rickmansworth.

Thomas, D. (1952) *Collected Poems 1934–1952*, Dent, London.

Thompson, F. (1996) *Where is dead? Children's questions about death*, unpublished MSc dissertation, University of Southampton.

Thompson, J. and Filshie, J. (1993) Transcutaneous nerve stimulation (TENS) and acupuncture, in *Oxford Textbook of Palliative Medicine* (eds D. Doyle, G. Hanks, N. Macdonald), Oxford University Press, Oxford.

Thorpe, G. (1993) Enabling more dying people to remain at home. *British Medical Journal*, **307**, 915–18.

Tobin, S. (1991) *Personhood in Advanced Old Age*, Springer, New York.

Townsend, J., Frank, A.O., Fermont, D., Dyer, S., Karran, O. and Walgrave, A. (1990) Terminal cancer and patients' preference for place of death. *British Medical Journal*, **301**, 415–17.

Townsend, P. (1962) *The Last Refuge*, Routledge, London.

T.R.S. (1856) The dream, in *The Child's Own Magazine for 1856* (1993) reprinted in *Death, Dying and Bereavement* (eds D. Dickenson and M. Johnson), Sage, London.

Twigg, J. (1989) Models of carers: how do social care agencies conceptualise their relationship with informal carers? *Journal of Social Policy*, **18**, 53–66.

Twycross, R. and Lichter, I. (1993) The terminal phase, in *Oxford Textbook of Palliative Medicine* (eds D. Doyle, G. Hanks and N Macdonald), Oxford University Press, Oxford.

Vachon, M. (1987) *Occupational Stress in the Care of the Critically Ill, the Dying and the Bereaved*, Hemisphere, New York.

Vachon, M. (1988) Battle fatigue in hospice/palliative care, in *A Safer Death: Multidisciplinary Aspects of Terminal Care* (eds A. Gilmore and S. Gilmore), Plenum Press, New York.

Vachon, M. (1995) Staff stress in hospice and palliative care: a review. *Palliative Medicine*, **9**, 91–122.

Van der Niet, L. (1995) *The perception of the nurse regarding the meaning of hope in terminally ill people and their role in helping to maintain hope*, unpublished MSc dissertation, University of Southampton.

Walker, J., Akinsanja, J.A., Davies, B.D. and Marcer, D. (1990) The nursing management of elderly patients with pain in the community. *Journal of Advanced Nursing*, **15**, 1154–61.

Walter, T. (1994) *The Revival of Death*, Routledge, London.

Walter, T. (1996) A new model of grief, *Mortality*, **1**, 7–25.

Webber, J. (1987) Accountability, advocacy and the nurse. *Palliative Medicine*, **1**, 53–6.

Webber, J. (1994) The evolving role of the Macmillan Nurse. *Nursing Times*, **90**(25), 66.

Weisman, A. (1972) *On Dying and Denying. A Psychiatric Study of Terminality*, Behavioural Publications, New York.

Weisman, A. and Kastenbaum, R. (1968) *The Psychological Autopsy: a Study of the Terminal Phase of Life*. Community Mental Health Monographs No. 4, Behavioural Publications, New York.

Weiss, R. (1991) The attachment bond in childhood and adulthood, in *Attachment across the Lifecycle* (eds C.M. Parkes, J. Stevenson-Hinde and P. Marris), Routledge, London.

Weiss, S.J. (1988) Touch, in *Annual Review of Nursing Research*, **6**, 3–27.

West, T. (1990) Multidisciplinary Working, in *Hospice and Palliative Care: an inter-disciplinary approach* (ed. C. Saunders), Edward Arnold, London.

West, T. (1993) The work of the interdisciplinary team, in *The Management of Terminal Malignant Disease* (eds C. Saunders and N. Sykes), Edward Arnold, London.

Wilkes, E. (1981) General Practitioner in a hospice. *British Medical Journal*, **282**, 1591.

Wilkes, E. (1993) Characteristics of hospice bereavement services. *Journal of Cancer Care*, **2**, 183–9.

Wilkinson, S. (1991) Factors which influence how nurses communicate with cancer patients. *Journal of Advanced Nursing*, **16**, 677–88.

Woodward, C.A. and King, B. (1993) Survivor Focus Groups: a quality assurance technique. *Palliative Medicine*, **7**, 229–34.

Worden. J.W. (1982) *Grief Counselling and Grief Therapy: A Handbook for the Mental Health Practitioner*, Springer, New York.

Worden, J.W. (1991) *Grief Counselling and Grief Therapy: A Handbook for the Mental Health Professional*, 2nd edn, Springer, New York.

World Health Organization (1990) *Cancer Pain Relief and Palliative Care*. Technical Report Services 804, World Health Organization, Geneva.

Wortman, C. and Silver, R.C. (1989) The myths of coping with loss. *Journal of Consulting and Clinical Psychology*, **57**, 349–57.

Wortman, C., Silver, R.O. and Kessler, R.C. (1993) Adjustment to bereavement, in *Handbook of Bereavement: theory, practice and intervention* (eds M.S. Stroebe, W. Stroebe and R.O. Hansson), University of Cambridge Press, Cambridge.

Wright, P. (1996) *Psychosexual dysfunction in women with gynaecological cancer receiving radiotherapy and their management by healthcare professionals*, unpublished MSc dissertation, University of Southampton.

Young, M., Benjamin, B. and Wallis, C. (1963) Mortality of widowers. *Lancet*, **ii**, 454.

Index

Advance directives 47
Advocacy 117
Anger 32, 54, 55
  working with anger 65–6
The arts in palliative care 128–31
Autonomy 59, 60, 114, 126
  in Netherlands 48
  patient's responsibility 25
  principle of 6, 7–8, 63

Behaviour therapy
  in profound grief 106
  in spiritual distress 33
Bereavement 90–107
  anticipatory grief 97
  around the death 100–1
  children 97, 103–5
  difficult problems 106–7
  and gender 94–5
  intervention 99, 102–3
  older people 97, 105
  pathological grief 98–9
  people with learning disabilities
    104, 105
  risk assessment 102
  risk factors 96–8
  stigmatised deaths 97–8, 105
  suicide 97, 106–7
  theory 91–6
    challenges 92–5
    development 91–2
    new approaches 95–6
  volunteers 103

Cancer Relief Macmillan Fund 38,
  41
  see also NSCR

Carers 1, 6, 9, 136
  conflicting demands 72–3
  and denial 63
  family meetings 86–7
  gender 72
  nature of family 71–2
  perceptions 76–7
  protective 80–1
  support for 50, 74–5
  views on treatment 46
Children
  after bereavement 103–5
  before bereavement 77–8, 82–6
Cognitive therapy 33, 60, 66
Complementary therapies 131
Communication 6, 8, 80–1, 136
  around the death 100–1
  breaking bad news 61–2
  confused older people 105
  with dying people 58–60
  non-verbal 60
  people with learning disabilities
    104, 105
  in teams 115–6
  value 33
  see also resolving conflict, denial,
    anger
Cultural attitudes
  autonomy 8
  bereavement 93–4
  body 19–20
  communication 59
  complementary therapies 131–2
  death 19, 21–2, 56, **fig 2.1**
  denial 57
  food 20
  illness 19

role of family 20, 71
staff stress 108
Culture 17–23
  definition 17
  migration 18

Death
  at home 49–52
  the last days 88–89
  moderm 21, 22
  neomodern 21–2
  in old age 14, 25–6, 29, 54
  psychological responses to 53–7
    "stages" 54–5, 56
    task approach 55
  taboo 21
  traditional 21
  at a young age 14, 26–7
Denial 25, 54, 55
  assessment 62
  and carers 63
  intervention 63–4
  and professionals 62–3
  theoretical issues 56–7
Depression 54, 66–7, *table 4.1*

Ethical issues
  access to palliative care 27–9
  communication 59, 60–1
  confused older people 105
  equity 12–3
  teamwork 116
  treatment 45–7
  see also autonomy, euthanasia
Euthanasia 36, 47–9
  see also autonomy

Genograms 79–80
Groups
  bereaved adults 99, 103
  bereaved children 104–5
  patients 69–70
  staff 120, 121–3

Help the hospices 39
Holistic approach 6, 9, 51, 52, 53, 126
  see also complementary therapies
Hope 24–5, 33
  see also spiritual care
Hospices
  changing work patterns 42
  establishment of St Christopher's
    36–7

growth 39
meaning of term 41
mixed economy of care 39–40
see also palliative care

Kuebler-Ross, Elisabeth 37, 53–4, 55,
  56, 93

Life review 32, 67–8

Macmillan nurses 38, 39, 111
Marie Curie Foundation 37, 38–9

National Society for Cancer Relief
  (NSCR) 37–8
National Council for Hospice and
  Specialist Palliative Care
  Services (NCHSPCS) 6, 34, 40,
  136

Palliative approach 6, 136
Palliative care
  access 27–9
  AIDS/HIV 42, 76, 90, 131
  arts 128–31
  continuing care 42–3, 136
  definitions 5–6
  development 35–40
  education 119–20
  future trends 40–4
  and gender 43–4, 72
  home care 48, 49–52
  outside cancer 41–2, 48, 136
  principles 6, 7–9, 136
  spread 44
  support teams 38, 40, 42, 136
  teamwork 112
  volunteers 113
  see also hospices
Psychosocial palliative care
  key concepts
    attachment 11, 36, 85, 91
    equity 11, 13–4, 27–9
    loss 11, 88, 95
    meaning 11, 12–3, 53, 126, 130
  who delivers 10

Quality assurance 133–5
  audit 134
  focus group 135
  perspective of dying person 134
Quality of life 6, 8, 41, 52, 57–8,
  136

Reminiscence 68
Resolving conflict
  cultural issues 29–31
  in families 86–7
  in teams 123–5

Saunders, Dame Cicely 13, 36–7, 40, 44
St Christopher's Hospice 13, 36, 37
Sexual issues 75–6, 81–2
Social support 73, 79, 85, 98, 110
Specialist palliative care services 6,
    42, 48, 116, 136
Spiritual issues 23–7
  care 31–4
  distress 32, 67, 110
  research 23–4
  terminal anguish 32
  who delivers 33–4
  see also anger, depression, hope
Staff stress 108–12
  prevention 127–9, 132, **fig 7.1**
  sources of stress 109–11

environment 110
  personal 109
Support systems 120–21

Teamwork 112–25
  education for 119–20
  effectiveness 112
  leadership 116, 118
  membership 113–5
  resolving conflict 123–5
  team building 117–9
Terminal care 6
Total pain 9, 10, 37, 55

Values
  empathy 15
  genuineness 15
  self-awareness 15
  self-determination 15
Volunteers
  bereavement 103
  palliative care 113